Diagnosis and Management of Complications of Peritoneal Dialysis related Peritonitis

Georgi Abraham • Santosh Varughese
Uma Sekar
Editors

Diagnosis and Management of Complications of Peritoneal Dialysis related Peritonitis

Springer

Editors
Georgi Abraham
Department of Nephrology
MGM Healthcare Chennai
Chennai, India

Santosh Varughese
Department of Nephrology
Christian Medical College and Hospital
Vellore, India

Uma Sekar
Department of Microbiology
Sri Ramachandra Medical College and
Research Institute
Chennai, India

ISBN 978-981-99-2277-2 ISBN 978-981-99-2275-8 (eBook)
https://doi.org/10.1007/978-981-99-2275-8

This Springer imprint is published by the registered company Springer Nature Singapore Pte Ltd.
The registered company address is: 152 Beach Road, #21-01/04 Gateway East, Singapore 189721, Singapore

Foreword

Many decades ago, it was reported that instillation of hypertonic solutions into the peritoneal cavity could effect osmotically induced fluid removal and could serve as a temporary treatment for congestive heart failure refractory to diuretics until a more definitive cardiac procedure could be undertaken. At this point, there was no realization that peritoneal dialysis could serve as a chronic therapy for maintenance dialysis in chronic kidney disease.

While the procedure did indeed lead to ultrafiltration, the incidence of peritonitis was so high that the infectious complications essentially replaced the complications of heart failure, leading to unchanged rates of hospitalization.

With the advent of maintenance PD, in the form of continuous ambulatory peritoneal dialysis (CAPD), the problem of peritonitis remained. Hospital wards were filled with PD patients suffering from this complication, and many patients at best had to transition to maintenance haemodialysis (HD) and at worst suffered serious morbidity or death. The advent of intraperitoneal instillation of antibiotics was a helpful advance, and protocols were devised to treat peritonitis this way. Nevertheless, the peritonitis rate remained high.

The advent of "flush before fill" was a major advance for PD. At the connection of the PD catheter to the dialysis bag, even with the most careful sterile technique, there is a risk of contamination of the connection site, particularly with ambient Gram-positive organisms. The connection procedure up to this point was that, after the connection (and possible contamination) the dialysis fluid flowed directly into the peritoneal cavity. With the double-bag flush before fill technique, however, while there was the same risk of inoculation of the connection with bacteria, the residing effluent was drained out of the peritoneal cavity into an empty drain bag and, for good measure, a small aliquot of fresh dialysis was also flushed though the system into the drain bag. Therefore, any potentially contaminated dialysis ended up in the drain bag, and not in the patient. This new technique led to a dramatic reduction in the incidence of peritonitis caused by Gram positive bacteria. Many units started reporting peritonitis rates of one episode every 3–4 years, compared to every 3–4 months in the earlier days.

Despite this advance, peritonitis is still with us. According to recent studies, it remains the principal cause of technique failure and sadly is still associated with high rates of morbidity and mortality. The book *Diagnosis and Management of Complications of Peritoneal Dialysis-related Peritonitis* will serve as an important companion to those around the world who are looking after PD patients. Encompassing both paediatric and adult patients, this book addresses all aspects on the prevention and treatment of peritonitis and the approach to complications, such as malnutrition and, of course, death.

I am sure we all look forward to the day when technical advances in the therapy will render this kind of educational material redundant, but for now this book will serve as an important resource in the care of our PD patients.

University of Toronto
Toronto, Canada

Joanne M. Bargman

Preface

Chronic Peritoneal Dialysis is an accepted therapy. However, there are many unmet needs and challenges we encounter in our practice. Infective complications leading to morbidity is a formidable challenge including PD-related peritonitis and increased patient fallout. This book with 13 chapters which are contributed by eminent nephrologists, ID experts, nutritionist, radiologist and pathologist provide interesting case reports, images, literature review and important take away points which is unique in presentation. The reader will learn and augment their knowledge base for practical applications in day-to-day practice.

Peritonitis can be a simple treatable and curable condition to be refractory and non-curable leading to catheter loss and subsequent high mortality in a subset of patients. Keeping this in mind the contributors have lucidly explained different aspects.

We would like to salute late Dr. Stephen Vas, Dr. Dimitrios G Oreopoulos and the thousands of patients who gave us immense knowledge about peritoneal dialysis.

We dedicate this book to our spouse's Rene, Rena, Sekar.

Chennai, India — Georgi Abraham
Chennai, India — Uma Sekar
Vellore, India — Santhosh Varughese

Contents

Prevention of Peritoneal Dialysis Related Infections Lessons to Learn

1

Maithrayie Kumaresan, Priyanka Govindhan,
Georgi Abraham, and Milly Mathew

60 years old male with DKD on CAPD, 2 L*3 exchanges of dextrose bags a day, presented with recurrent episodes of lower GI bleed for the previous 2 weeks. His dialysis effluent was clear. After GI consult a colonoscopy was suggested. As per ISPD guidelines, patient received prophylactic antibiotics—single dose IP 15 mg/kg cefazolin plus 0.6 mg/kg gentamycin in the previous exchange and emptying the peritoneal cavity was carried out to prevent the onset of peritonitis.

1.1 Introduction

Peritoneal dialysis (PD) related infections continue to be a serious complication for CAPD patients. CAPD and APD are two modes of peritoneal dialysis therapy all over the world using permanent peritoneal dialysis access implanted by either a bed side technique, open surgery or laparoscopic methods by a trained person, a nephrologist or a surgeon. CAPD catheter insertion-related peritonitis is defined as the episode of peritonitis that occurs within 30 days of PD catheter insertion. The risk for peritonitis commences from the first day of CAPD training and is prevalent throughout the course of dialysis, regardless of the setting. Peritonitis can be associated with abdominal pain, hospitalization, catheter loss, transfer to hemodialysis as well as a risk of death [1]. On the other hand, enteric causes of peritonitis pose a diagnostic difficulty ending up in delayed treatment and increased mortality rates [2].

M. Kumaresan
University Hospital Lewisham, London, UK

P. Govindhan
Nephrology Colorado University School of Medicine, Aurora, CO, USA

G. Abraham (✉) · M. Mathew
MGM Healthcare, Chennai, Tamil Nadu, India

G. Abraham et al. (eds.), *Diagnosis and Management of Complications of Peritoneal Dialysis related Peritonitis*,
https://doi.org/10.1007/978-981-99-2275-8_1

Prevention of peritoneal dialysis related peritonitis is the primary objective of learning, training and application to all personal involved in peritoneal dialysis.

1.2 Gut Microbiota and Procedure Related Peritonitis

Under normal physiological conditions, swallowed bacteria from the oral cavity or the upper respiratory tract are lodged in the upper gastro-intestinal tract and remain at low bacterial counts $<10^5$ colony-forming units (CFU/mL) whereas the colon bacterial counts usually exceed 10^9 CFU/mL. An absence of normal colonic flora is associated with reductions in mucosal cell turnover, vascularity, muscle wall thickness, motility, baseline cytokine production and defective cell-mediated immunity [2].

Endoscopically assisted invasive procedures, such as biopsy, polypectomy, intrauterine device implantation/removal, and dilatation and curettage, pose a high risk for peritonitis. The prevalence of upper GIscopy (UGI)-associated peritonitis (1.2–3.9%) is in theory lower than colonoscopy (3.4–8.5%) or hysteroscopy (26.9–38.5%) -associated peritonitis [3]. Studies have also shown that histamine-2 receptor blocker consumption is associated with a higher rate of UGIscopy peritonitis (9.4%) compared to the control cohort (2.9%) [3]. The underlying effect can be attributed to the bactericidal effect of gastric juice. On the contrary, a copious amount of normal microflora in the vagina (10^5–10^8 CFU/mL) can ascend into the peritoneal cavity through the cervix during hysteroscopy, increasing the risk of the hysteroscopy-associated peritonitis. The transmural migration of bacteria into the peritoneal cavity during UGIscopy is hindered by a greater mural thickness and a shorter bowel segment. Hence, prophylactic antibiotic- single dose oral 2 g amoxicillin one hour prior to dental procedures is recommended for peritonitis prevention.

1.3 Special Situations to Prevent Peritonitis

1. Proud flesh tissue develops at the exit site of the catheter as described above in a 65-year old man on CAPD over 1 year. It was not related to trauma. The exact pathophysiology is not known. However, it is an inflammatory lesion with redness. If the lesion is weepy a gram stain and culture should be sent before cauterization. Cauterization with 75% silver nitrate was done and the patient was instructed to do daily exit site care and mupirocin ointment along with ofloxacin PO 400 mg OD for 7 days. Proud flesh if infected can lead to exit site and tunnel infection leading to peritonitis and catheter loss (Figs. 1.1 and 1.2).
2. Relocation of the exit site

We describe a 7 years old boy with CATKUT on CAPD using a double cuff swan neck Tenckhoff paediatric catheter. After 11 months he developed exit site infection with proud flesh tissue which grew Pseudomonas Aeruginosa. He was treated with Cefotaxime and cauterization with silver nitrate [3]. Nine months later he had a

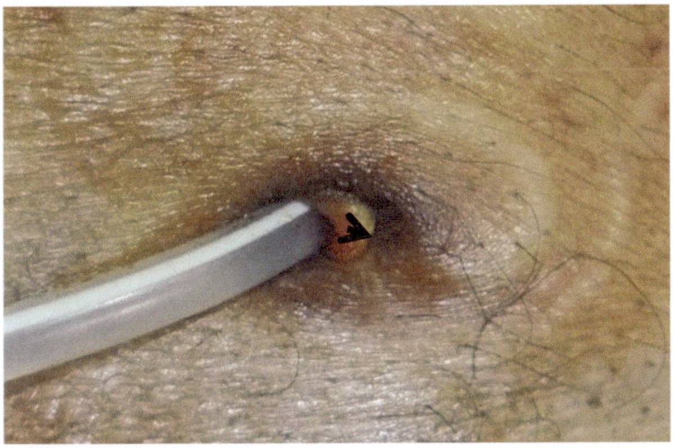

Fig. 1.1 Proud flesh with inflammation

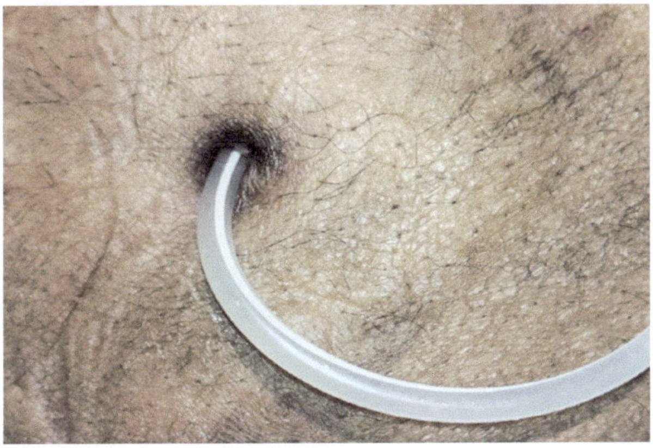

Fig. 1.2 Proud flesh after 1 week of silver nitrate cauterization

second episode of exit site infection with the distal cuff migrating to the exit site (Figs. 1.3 and 1.4) with pain and tenderness. Culture yeilded *Pseudomonas Aeruginosa* which was not responding to the antibiotic regimen. As the infection was refractory, deroofing of the tunnel and cuff shaving was done. The tunnel and catheter werewashed with betadine and antibiotic solution. The catheter was bought out through a new tunnel (Figs. 1.3 and 1.4).

This led to resolution of infection and prolonged the life of the catheter, thereby preventing catheter loss and effective long-term solution for chronic exit site infection.

3. CAPD in Ureterostomy patients

A 3-year-old male baby weighing 10 kgs with Congenital Abnormality of Kidney Urinary Tract (CAKUT) was initiated on CAPD. He was on 500 cc of dialysate four times a day. In Fig. 1.5, a functioning ureterostomy which was discharging urine on the left side and right-side ureterostomy was closed previously. The presence of nephrostomy should not deter one from providing chronic peritoneal dialysis. The

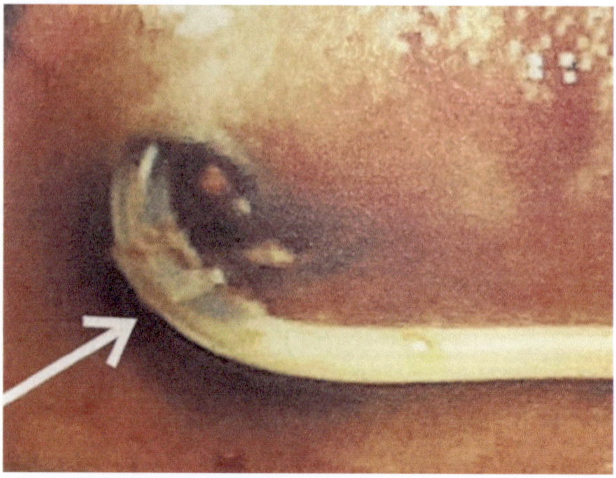

Fig. 1.3 Infected distal dacron cuff with deroofing and cuff shaving

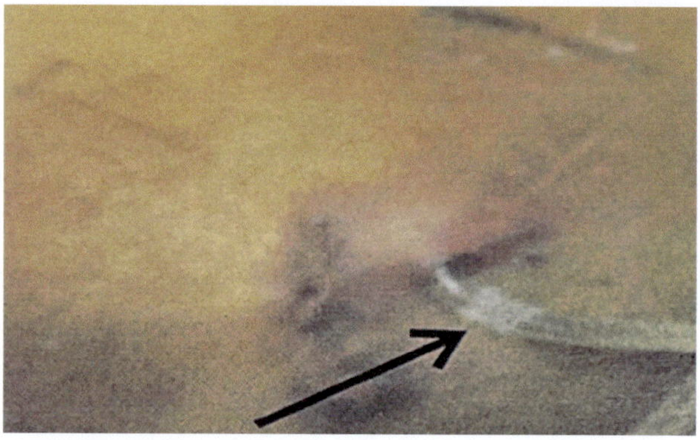

Fig. 1.4 Shaved cuff with healed exit site and relocation

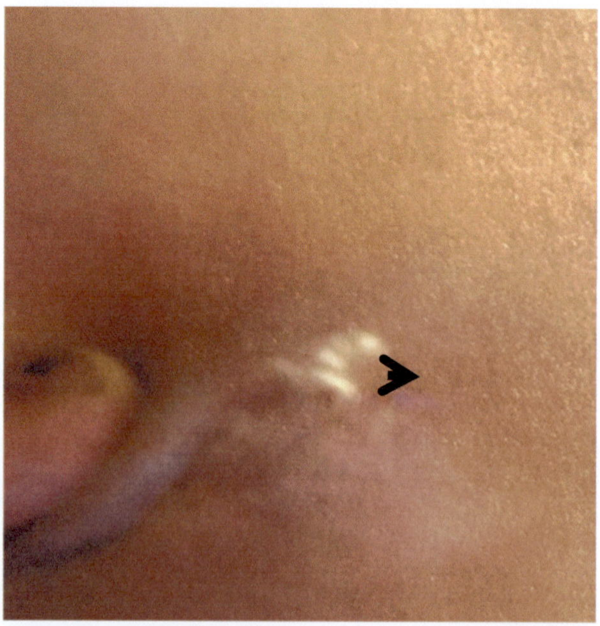

Fig. 1.5 Dribbling urine from the ureterostomy site

exchanges need to be performed with precaution to prevent contamination from the urine coming out of the nephrostomy site. He was on Tab cefaclor 2.5 mg HS. Prevention of peritoneal catheter related infections in children include avoidance of pull and torsion of the catheter, daily exit site catheter, prompt treatment of upper respiratory infections and appropriate use of antibiotics with congenital anomalies of genitourinary tract.

4. Catheter damage—An avoidable cause for peritonitis

Sharp objects should not be accidentally brought to the catheter surface as this may lead to nick in the catheter leading to dialysate leak and peritonitis. Rarely, spontaneous catheter rupture can occur leading to dialysate leak. The leak should be recognised immediately and the catheter proximal to the leak should be clamped. In case of catheter rupture (Fig. 1.6), the catheter maybe saved by using available catheter length connected to the non-damaged portion by a titanium adaptor, thereby, conserving the catheter. Antibiotic prophylaxis as in peritonitis should be implemented and fluid should be checked for cloudiness and abdominal pain.

Safety pins are sometimes used to maintain the grip of clothes by patients. This may inadvertently pierce the catheter producing multiple holes which cannot be sealed. This will lead to peritonitis due to contamination. Examination of the catheter will show multiple water leakage points as in one of our patients who was on CAPD for 2 years (Fig. 1.7). Patient should be advised strictly against sharp instruments in the vicinity of the catheter to prevent contamination related peritonitis (Fig. 1.8).

Ultrasound examination of the catheter tunnel is an important tool for diagnosing tunnel infection and early treatment to prevent development of peritonitis and catheter loss. Follow up ultrasound during anti-microbial therapy is helpful in response to treatment. The presence of tunnel infection with peritonitis requires anti-microbial therapy and catheter removal for cure.

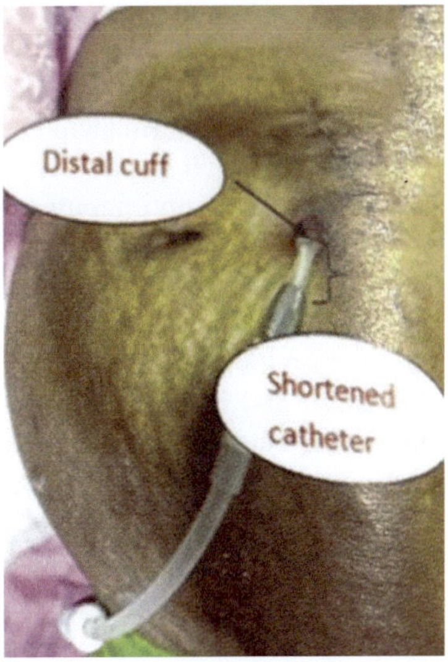

Fig. 1.6 Catheter rupture sites

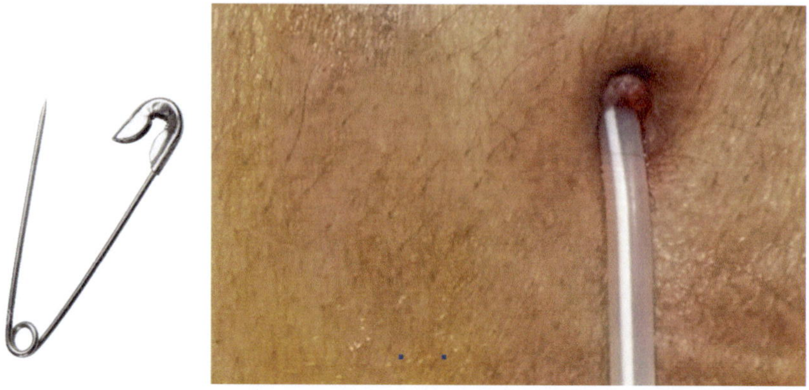

Fig. 1.7 PD catheter pierced by safety pin

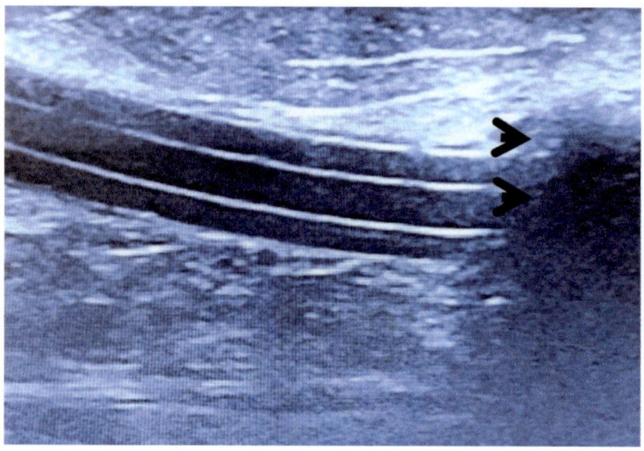

Fig. 1.8 Catheter and tunnel in a patient post peritonitis, post-implantation showing absence of collection ensuring safety of PD

1.4 Prevention of PD Related Peritonitis

Catheter selection and placement: Early post implantation infection is prevented by choosing the right permanent catheter site of implantation either through the anterior abdominal wall or pre-sternal region. A swan neck double dacron cuff catheter should be used for optimal ingrowth and fixation. The proximal cuff holds the catheter in place and the distal cuff acts as a barrier to prevent infection. Total aseptic precautions should be ensured, ideal placement of the tip of the catheter in to the bony pelvis ensuring appropriate in and out flow of sterile dialysis fluid, creation of a downward looking exit site, sterilization of the anterior abdominal wall using sprit or betadine and proper catheter immobilization to be followed. Studies have proved that coiled catheters do better than straight catheters in terms of minimizing tip migration (drainage failure) and have better catheter survival [1] The introduction of Y set for PD has dramatically reduced the rate of peritonitis due to less contamination in comparison to the straight spike system. APD being a therapy with single connection and disconnect system has also ensured reduction in peritonitis due to touch contamination compared to CAPD.

Pre and post procedure prophylaxis: Prophylactic antibiotic therapy within 1 h of the procedure by intravenous vancomycin 1 gm or first/second generation cephalosporins should be administered. Use of antibiotic cream at the exit site- either mupirocin to prevent gram positive infections or gentamicin cream to prevent gram positive and gram-negative infections, avoidance of mechanical stress on the exit site - reduces the occurrence of exit site infections and peritonitis. CAPD patients should be asked about pets during training and home visits or after a diagnosis of unusual organisms suspicious of zoonoses because peritonitis due to zoonotic organisms can occur in the context of close contact with companion animals.

Surgical Technique: Laparoscopic or open surgical techniques are preferred for catheter placement. The laparoscopic technique offers an advantage in this regard due to direct visualization of the peritoneal cavity and easy lysis of prior adhesions. The exit site and the intra-peritoneal tip of the catheter should not be sutured as this may cause an exit site infection or catheter movement. The catheter can be capped after the peritoneal cavity is flushed with 500 to 1500 ml of heparinized dialysate until the effluent becomes clear. The exit site and surgical incision are covered with sterile gauze and a non-occlusive dressing. The patient is advised to minimize contact with the catheter and surgical incisions until the wounds have healed and the tunnel has matured. The catheter is taped securely and remains immobile for 2 weeks to ensure adequate healing. Beginning PD before the deep cuff matures increases the risk of leakage [4]. A low volume exchange should be performed to assess the patency of the catheter before moving on to high volume exchanges.

Prevention of mechanical stress at exit site: Pre-procedure Foleys catheter insertion is crucial to prevent retention of urine and to aid early detection of improper catheter insertion. Avoidance of constipation by emptying the bowels through soap and water enemas to prevent migration of catheter tip.

Anterior nares culture: As a common practice individuals touch inside or outside of the nostrils and can be carriers of staphylococcus either methicillin sensitive Staph Aureus (MSSA) or Methicillin resistance Staph Aureus (MRSA) which can break the aseptic technique leading to gram positive peritonitis. Hence an anterior nares swabs of the patient and attender is mandatory before starting the training for either of them. At least 3 swabs must be taken with proper aseptic techniques. Screening for nasal carriers and gingivitis and proactive treatment- intranasal calcium preparation of mupirocin in a liquid paraffin base twice/day for 5-7 days reduces the emergence of exit site and tunnel infections. In resistant cases, either oral rifampicin 600 mg OD may be useful.

Dry and wet contamination: When patients report contamination during an exchange procedure, the need for treatment is driven by distinguishing 'dry contamination' -contamination outside a closed PD system, such as disconnection distal to a closed clamp from 'wet contamination' -referring to contamination with an open system, when either dialysis fluid is infused after contamination or if the catheter administration set has been left open for an extended period. Examples of wet contamination include leaks from dialysate bags, leaks or breaks in tubing proximal to the tubing clamp, breach of aseptic technique or touch contamination of the connection during a PD exchange. Prophylactic antibiotics is only recommended after wet contamination. A PD effluent should preferably be obtained for cell count and culture after wet contamination. A wet contamination should be monitored closely for an extended period, as a broader spectrum of organisms might lead to peritonitis.

1.5 Important Points

- All attempts should be made to prevent occurrence of peritonitis in PD patients.
- Prophylactic antimicrobialtherapy must be given to CAPD patients undergoing upper and lower GI endoscopy.
- Extreme caution should be exercised in preventing exit site infection with appropriate exit site care.
- Catheter damage should be prevented by cautions handling of the permanent catheter.
- Pre implantation antibiotic prophylaxis and preparation including skin preparation bowel enema should be advocated.

References

1. Bender FH, Bernardini J, Piraino B. Prevention of infectious complications in peritoneal dialysis: best demonstrated practices. Kidney Int Suppl. 2006;103:S44–54. https://doi.org/10.1038/sj.ki.5001915.
2. Kern EO, Newman LN, Cacho CP, Schulak JA, Weiss MF. Abdominal catastrophe revisited: the risk and outcome of enteric peritoneal contamination. Perit Dial Int. 2002;22(3):323–34. https://doi.org/10.1177/089686080202200305.
3. Tan SY, Thiruventhiran T. Catheter cuff shaving using a novel technique: a rescue treatment for persistent exit-site infections. Perit Dial Int. 2000;20(4):471–2. https://doi.org/10.1177/089686080002000417.
4. Gokal R, Ash SR, Helfrich GB, Holmes CJ, Joffe P, Nichols WK, Oreopoulos DG, Riella MC, Slingeneyer A, Twardowski ZJ, et al. Peritoneal catheters and exit-site practices: toward optimum peritoneal access. Perit Dial Int. 1993;13(1):29–39.

2 Preventing Peritonitis: Role of Nurses

Usha Jacob, G. Padma, and Reena Rachel George

Ms. S, a 9-year-old girl from Islampur, Bangladesh, lost her mother to ESKD when she was only 3 years old. In October 2021, when she developed renal calculi, with occurrence of the same disease that affected her mother and progressing to ESKD requiring initiation of renal replacement therapy, her father was absolutely devastated. She was initiated on hemodialysis in Islampur with a brachiocephalic fistula as her vascular access. However, her father wishing that his daughter would be able to lead a more normal life, without intrusion to her studies and social activity, brought her to Christian Medical College Vellore to explore alternate options of treatment. A living kidney transplantation was not a viable option due to non-availability of related donors. The option of PD was explained to her father by the PD nurse educator. Her father, although initially hesitant considering the challenges of having to perform PD exchanges for his daughter 3 times a day, embraced the idea, understanding that the PD program will allow his daughter to attend regular classes at school and have a relatively normal life.

After further counselling and education, Ms. S underwent bedside percutaneous PD catheter insertion by a nephrologist and was initiated on 3 PD exchanges during the day and one night dwell with 2 L of 2.5% Dextrose. As done for all patients being initiated on PD, Ms. S received 3 weeks of training to perform PD exchange and exit site care on a mannequin and on herself under expert supervision of the PD nurse. Her father was taught troubleshooting in case of any PD-related complications that can be safely managed at home. A handbook with details of the procedure and troubleshooting tips in their own language was given to them.

U. Jacob · R. R. George (✉)
Christian Medical College Vellore, Vellore, Tamil Nadu, India

G. Padma
Tanker Foundation, Chennai, Tamil Nadu, India

G. Abraham et al. (eds.), *Diagnosis and Management of Complications of Peritoneal Dialysis related Peritonitis*,
https://doi.org/10.1007/978-981-99-2275-8_2

The father and daughter who were initially apprehensive and uncertain were now confident and competent to continue performing PD procedure at home. Ms. S and her father are instructed to tele consult the PD nurse educator in case of any difficulties that they encounter related to PD.

Now Ms. S is active with decreased symptoms of kidney failure and continuing to attend regular classes at school. There has not been any PD catheter-related infections or other complications thus far.

2.1 Introduction

In view of the chronic nature of the disease, patients with end-stage kidney disease (ESKD) may be best served if they can be motivated to manage their therapy themselves and thus be empowered to live a near normal, productive life with excellent quality of life. It is often a challenge for peritoneal dialysis (PD) nurse to tailor PD training to patients of varied cultural, ethnic, and educational backgrounds. Organizing and establishing an efficient PD program should be the combined effort of the nephrologist and PD nurse. An effective PD training provided by a committed, compassionate, and competent nurse coupled with consistent follow-up can significantly reduce the incidence of exit site infection, tunnel infection, and peritonitis. In the words of the late Professor Dr. Dimitrios G. Oreopoulos, "A well—informed and enthusiastic nurse is a great blessing to the nephrologists and the peritoneal dialysis patient." [1]

2.2 Peritonitis Prevention Strategies

1. *Selection of Patients* [2]

Patients for PD are to be selected carefully, assessing the level of motivation to learn and perform the procedure, and to strictly adhere to aseptic techniques and principles. The patient's selection of PD as their preferred modality always supersedes the physician's decision on behalf of the patient. A thorough history and physical examination is performed to identify/understand any contraindications to PD and to obtain baseline data about the patient. Patients must also have minimum facilities in their houses, school, or workplaces to have a designated, clean place to perform PD exchanges.

2. *Preparation for PD Catheter Insertion* [2]

The PD catheter may be inserted percutaneously under local anesthesia by the nephrologist or by laparotomy/laparoscopy by the surgeon depending on local practice. Information about the proposed procedure and modality should be provided to patients and their families in their own language, preferably by showing video clip/pictures of the procedure, thus allowing patient and family to make an informed decision and provide consent. The PD nurse must ensure that the patient is kept nil per oral for at least 6 h prior to the procedure to avoid infection. An intravenous dose of antibiotic (usually vancomycin or cefazolin) is administered prophylactically to reduce the incidence of catheter exit site colonization, wound infection, early exit site infection, and tunnel infection. Patient must be instructed to take povidone iodine scrub bath on the morning of the procedure and to wear the clean hospital gown provided.

The nurse must ensure that the procedure room surfaces are cleaned with 7% Lysol (or similar disinfectant), and in certain units, the air is sprayed with EcoShield (hydrogen peroxide preparation). The cleaning protocol may vary based on local practice in different facilities. The nurse may assist in PD catheter insertion and must ensure that the same is done using sterile equipment and adhering to aseptic techniques.

3. *Exit Site Care* [3]

After catheter placement, exit site should be kept dry, and patient is instructed to avoid taking direct shower or tub bath till wound healing take place. Handling of the catheter should be kept to a minimum to enhance the healing of exit wound. Cleaning of the exit site with normal saline after removal of dressing and bath is advised from the fifth day after PD catheter placement. Patients and relatives are taught to perform exit site care once daily using normal saline and sterile gauze to clean the site from around the catheter to outside in circular strokes. (Fig. 2.1) Patients are instructed to bathe before performing exit site care.

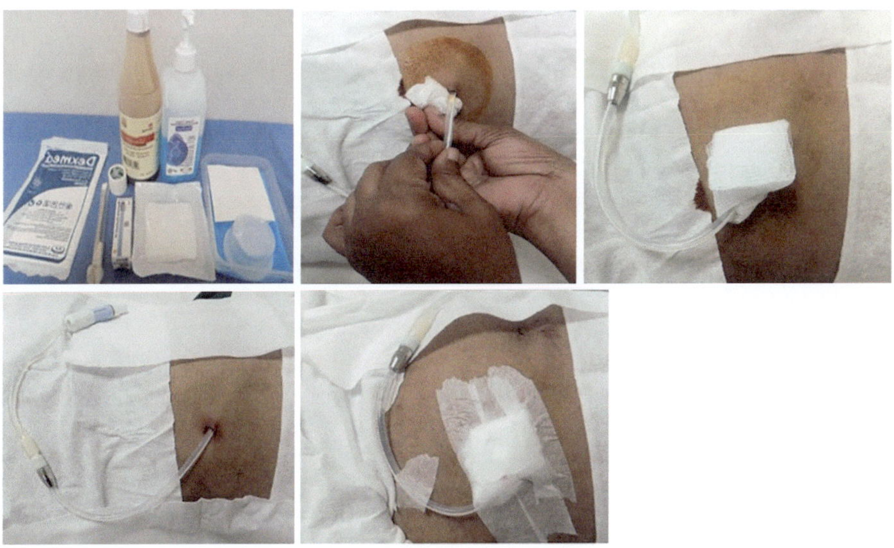

Fig. 2.1 Steps in exit site care (photographs taken by the author)

The exit site area is protected using a dry gauze. The catheter is coiled and kept in a cloth pouch which is secured around the waist with a Velcro belt. This avoids pulling on the catheter and exposure of superficial cuff and catheter to the outside. Immobilization of the catheter at the exit site is also emphasized.

Patients and families are to be taught to identify and report signs and/or symptoms of exit site infection, i.e., purulent discharge, redness, pain, swelling, and warmth around the exit site area. In case of any suggestion of an exit site infection, the PD nurse grades the exit site infection as 0, 1, 2, 3, or 4 grades, and the discharge from the site (if any) is collected and sent for gram stain, culture, and sensitivity. Prophylactic antibiotic therapy should be initiated (with concomitant anti-fungal prophylaxis). Antibiotics may need to be changed based on the culture and sensitivity reports.

A root cause analysis must be done by the PD nurse to identify any breach in technique or any faulty step that may have led to the exit site infection. PD exchange and exit site care training must be reinforced.

4. *Following Aseptic Techniques While Performing PD Exchanges* [3, 4]

After the break-in period (typically 2 weeks for surgically placed catheters and shorter for percutaneously inserted catheters), the patients and the caregivers are instructed to strictly adhere to the following practices that prevent peritonitis.

(i) Perform PD exchanges in a clean designated place.
(ii) Store PD supplies in a clean and dry place.
(iii) Check the PD fluid bag noting the expiry date and regularly look for color change, sediments, or leak.
(iv) Change the transducer set every 3 to 4 months.
(v) Perform hand hygiene following all the steps prior to each exchange.
(vi) Place a sterile towel beneath the catheter, on the abdomen prior to each exchange.
(vii) Use a sterile, small dressing pack and povidone iodine to clean the catheter cap before removing it.
(viii) Minimal touch technique to be followed throughout the exchange procedure.

5. *Prophylactic Antibiotic Therapy Before Procedures like Colonoscopy and Dental Procedures* [4]
6. *Nutritional Advice* [4]

Considering that the patients on PD lose protein, the patients are advised to take 1.3 to 1.5 g protein/kg/day. Low intake of protein can lead to low serum albumin and malnutrition making patients on PD susceptible to infection. The nurse instructs the patients to take a diet that is high in protein, vitamins, and iron. Nutrition is covered in detail elsewhere in the book.

7. *Early Identification of Peritonitis* [4]

The PD nurse must teach all the patients and the caregivers the identifying signs and symptoms of peritonitis:

(i) Fever
(ii) Cloudy PD drain fluid
(iii) Abdominal pain/tenderness
(iv) Vomiting

A diagnosis of peritonitis is confirmed with clinical findings accompanied by the culture report of PD fluid sample. PD fluid from the first bag of cloudy solution is collected adhering to protocol and sent for culture and sensitivity test. Empirical antibiotic therapy is initiated intraperitoneally by the PD nurse which is later changed based on antibiotic susceptibility. All patients are taught how to give antibiotic injections intraperitoneally maintaining a minimum dwell time of 2 h.

If identified early, peritonitis can often be treated appropriately with intraperitoneal antibiotic therapy, preserving the PD catheter. Antimicrobial therapy in discussed in detail elsewhere in the book.

Steps in Collecting PD Fluid Sample for Culture [5]
The steps of collecting the PD fluid sample are illustrated in Fig. 2.2:

(i) Wear a surgical mask.
(ii) Keep povidone-iodine, sterile syringe, and sterile gauze available.

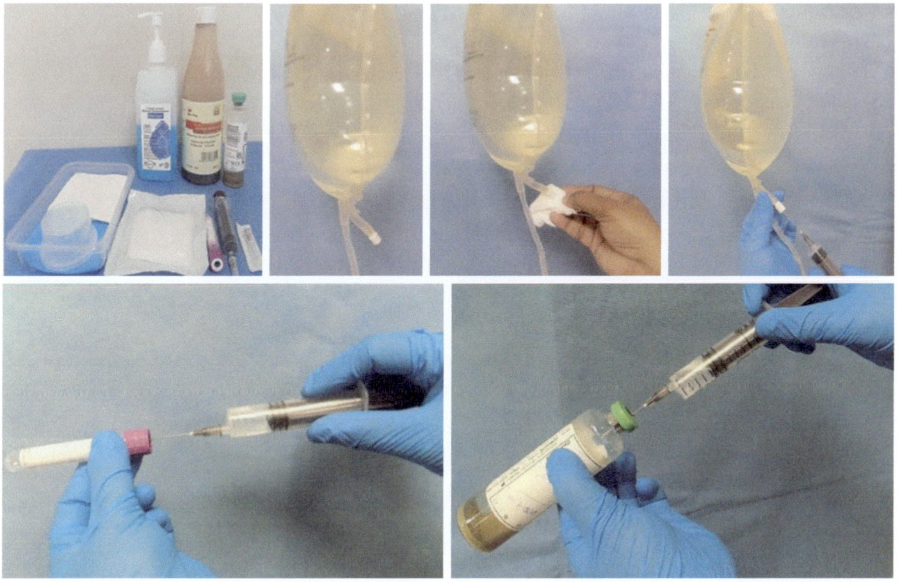

Fig. 2.2 Steps in collecting PD fluid sample for culture (photographs taken by the author)

(iii) Perform hand hygiene.
(iv) Medication port of dialysis bag is to be cleaned for 30 sec. with povidone-iodine solution and allowed to dry.
(v) Aspirate PD fluid with a sterile syringe and transfer it to the blood culture bottle and to the counts tube.
(vi) Alternatively, the entire bag of PD fluid may be sent to the laboratory for analysis.

Steps in Collecting Exit Site Swab Sample for Culture [5]

(i) Open swab pack using aseptic technique.
(ii) Prior to taking the culture, thoroughly cleanse the exit site with sterile water or saline. This provides moisture to the wound bed to improve the bacterial yield.
(iii) Remove excess water/saline using a sterile gauze.
(iv) Rotate tip of sterile swab over 1 cm^2 area of viable tissue for 5 seconds using sufficient pressure to extract underlying fluid from exit site. This ensures that the swab is collected from viable tissue and not necrotic, purulent material or eschar that is heavily contaminated with bacteria and may result in inaccurate culture results.
(v) Place swab stick into the tube with medium.
(vi) Apply dressing to the wound.
(vii) Label and send swab to laboratory as soon as possible. Transportation delays must be avoided as these may result in some bacteria dying, and others overgrown by more rapidly growing strains.

Steps in Instilling Antibiotics Intraperitoneally

(i) Wear a surgical mask.
(ii) Keep povidone-iodine, sterile syringe, sterile gauze available.
(iii) Perform hand hygiene.
(iv) Medication port of dialysis bag is to be cleaned for 30 sec. with povidone-iodine solution and allowed to dry.
(v) Load the required dose of medication in a syringe and administer through medication port and record the same.

8. *Self-Care* [4, 5]

Patients are taught to keep themselves clean and their surroundings neat and tidy. Healthy habits like avoidance of constipation and regular bathing are also encouraged.

2.3 Prevention of Future Episodes of Peritonitis [4, 5]

If a patient develops a peritonitis episode, apart from treating them adequately, a root cause analysis needs to be carried out to check if there was any break in technique or any action that could have been taken to prevent the peritonitis episode.

Retraining of the patient and caregiver after each peritonitis episode is also a vital part of preventing a future episode. Whenever there is a change in caregiver, training needs to be imparted formally to the new caregiver.

2.4 Conclusion

PD peritonitis is a common but potentially preventable complication of peritoneal dialysis. Efficient education and effective training of patients and caregivers by PD nurse are the key factors that minimizes complications associated with PD, especially peritonitis, the impact of which cannot be underestimated. Effective preventive strategies must be planned and implemented by the team that include the renal physician/nephrologist, PD nurse, nutritionist, and, most importantly, the patient and/or caregiver. Often, the risk factors for development of PD peritonitis are trivial but an ignored factor, which, if taken care of, can prevent PD peritonitis, and this will go a long way to boost the growth of peritoneal dialysis as a modality of choice of renal replacement therapy, dispelling the false sense of fear and anxiety associated with the option of peritoneal dialysis in prospective patients with ESKD.

2.5 Important Points

- The PD nurse is arguably the most important member of the treating team in preventing the occurrence of PD peritonitis.
- Patients for PD as are to be selected carefully with the patient's selection of PD as their preferred modality being preferred to the physician's choice.
- Patients are taught exit site care, immobilization of the catheter, and aseptic techniques while performing PD exchanges.
- Patients are taught to recognize early the occurrence of PD peritonitis if it occurs so that antibiotics can be started promptly.
- Needs for prophylactic antibiotics before procedures, appropriate self-care, and advice on nutrition are other aspects of PD education that the PD nurse imparts.
- If/when a PD peritonitis episode does occur, the onus is on the PD nurse to do root cause analysis and to take corrective action including retraining of patient and caregiver after each peritonitis episode. Equally crucial is to impart formal training if/whenever there is a change in caregiver.

References

1. Oreopoulos DG. The peritoneal dialysis nurse: the key to success. Perit Dial Bull. 1981;1:113–4.
2. Crabtree JH, Hathaway PB. Patient selection and planning for image-guided peritoneal dialysis catheter placement. Semin Intervent Radiol. 2022;39(1):32–9.
3. Figueiredo AE, Bernardini J, Bowes E, Hiramatsu M, Price V, Su C, Walker R, Brunier G. A syllabus for teaching peritoneal dialysis to patients and caregivers. Perit Dial Int. 2016;36(6):592–605. https://doi.org/10.3747/pdi.2015.00277.

4. Li PK-T, Chow KM, Cho Y, et al. ISPD peritonitis guideline recommendations: 2022 update on prevention and treatment. Perit Dial Int. 2022;42(2):110–53.
5. Li PK, Szeto CC, Piraino B, de Arteaga J, Fan S, Figueiredo AE, Fish DN, Goffin E, Kim YL, Salzer W, Struijk DG, Teitelbaum I, Johnson DW. ISPD peritonitis recommendations: 2016 update on prevention and treatment. Perit Dial Int. 2016;36(5):481–508.

Peritonitis-Free Peritoneal Dialysis Initiation in ICU on Urgent Basis: It Is Possible

3

P. Bavikar, P. K. Etta, R. Jasti, S. Antony, L. Pradhan, and K. S. Nayak

3.1 Clinical Vignette

48-year-old male, Mr. GS, presented with fever, abdominal distension, pedal edema, and reduced urine output since 5 days. There was no history of hematuria, dysuria, foul smelling urine, abdominal tenderness, and passage of fleshy mass during micturition. He is known case of hypertension and type 2 diabetes mellitus. There was no history of stroke, coronary artery disease, and NSAID abuse in the past. His weight was 109 kgs, height 178 cm, and BMI 34.4 kg/m^2. His pulse was 88/min; BP was 90/60 mmHg.

His relevant laboratory investigations were as follows:

Hemoglobin—8.8 gm/dl
platelet count—3.08 lakhs/cumm
Urea—131 mg/dl
Creatinine—7.92 mg/dl
APTT—36.5 secs
INR—1.0

He was admitted in ICU and started on inotropic supports. Bedside PD catheter (42 cm Tenckhoff catheter) was inserted in the midline 5 cm infra-umbilically and subcutaneous, tunnel was made 5 cm lateral to the catheter insertion site. 24 h later automated peritoneal dialysis was initiated with 2 bags of 5 L–1.5% PD fluid bags. Patient tolerated peritoneal dialysis for the next 10 days. He was clinically and hemodynamically better with treatment.

P. Bavikar · P. K. Etta · R. Jasti · S. Antony · L. Pradhan · K. S. Nayak (✉)
Virinchi Hospita, Hyderabad, Telangana, India

G. Abraham et al. (eds.), *Diagnosis and Management of Complications of Peritoneal Dialysis related Peritonitis*,
https://doi.org/10.1007/978-981-99-2275-8_3

3.2 Introduction

Patients with "dialysis-requiring-AKI" are critical and require intensive care unit (ICU) admission. Dialysis requiring AKI is invariably treated with hemodialysis (HD) or hemofiltration. Although multiple studies have shown the efficacy of peritoneal dialysis in AKI, it is under-utilized in the critical setting [1, 2]. Peritoneal dialysis (PD) associated peritonitis (PDAP) is a major complication, leading to its hesitant use in the acute setting. However, it cannot be denied that patients on hemodialysis too are at risk of catheter-related blood stream infections (CRBSI). Hence, PD should not be discounted as a modality for renal replacement therapy in critically ill.

3.3 Definitions

Conventionally, PD is initiated after 14 days of peritoneal dialysis catheter insertion. Urgent start PD (*USPD*) is defined as use of peritoneal dialysis catheter within 14 days of insertion [3].

Emergent start PD (*ESPD*) implies starting PD immediately on presentation, with APD being initiated once PD catheter is inserted [4].

The ISPD peritonitis guidelines 2022 defines *PD catheter insertion-related peritonitis* as an episode of peritonitis that occurs within 30 days of PD catheter insertion and should be <5% of PD catheter insertions [5].

The *break-in period* refers to the time between catheter insertion and routine catheter use. The treatment strategy used during the break-in period allows patients to adapt to the dialysis process.

Dwell time implies the duration of time; the dialysate solution remains in the abdomen. The time between dialysate solution instillation to removal is dwell time.

Dry contamination is contamination outside a closed PD system, such as disconnection distal to a closed clamp.

Wet contamination refers to contamination with an open system, when either dialysis fluid is infused after contamination or if the catheter administration set has been left open for an extended period.

An *Exchange* is the process of filling and then draining dialysate solute from the abdomen.

Types of PD initiation based on break-in period (Fig. 3.1)

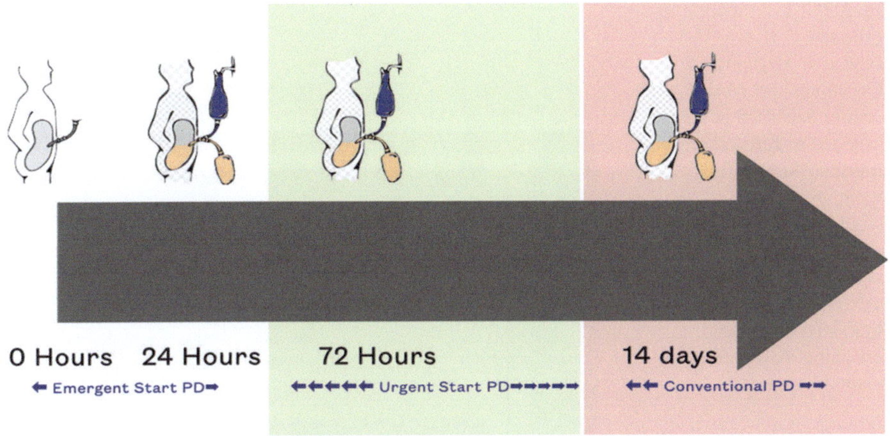

Fig. 3.1 Peritoneal Dialysis (PD) Terminologies based on timing of catheter placement (0 h) and PD initiation (24 hours, 48 hours, 72 hours, 14 days). (PD - Peritoneal dialysis, ESPD - Emergent Start Peritoneal Dialysis, USPD - Urgent Start Peritoneal Dialysis)

3.4 What Is PDAP?

Peritoneal dialysis-associated peritonitis encompasses PD-related peritonitis and PD catheter-related infections (exit site infection (ESI) and tunnel infection) [5].

ISPD 2022 guidelines [5] recommends diagnosing peritonitis in the presence of at least 2 of the following criteria:

1. Abdominal pain and/or cloudy dialysis effluent
2. Dialysis effluent white cell count >100/μL or > 0.1 × 10^9/L (after a dwell time of at least 2 h), with >50% polymorphonuclear leukocytes (PMN)
3. Positive dialysis effluent culture

The classification of peritonitis (adapted from ISPD peritonitis guideline recommendations: 2022) is illustrated in Fig. 3.2

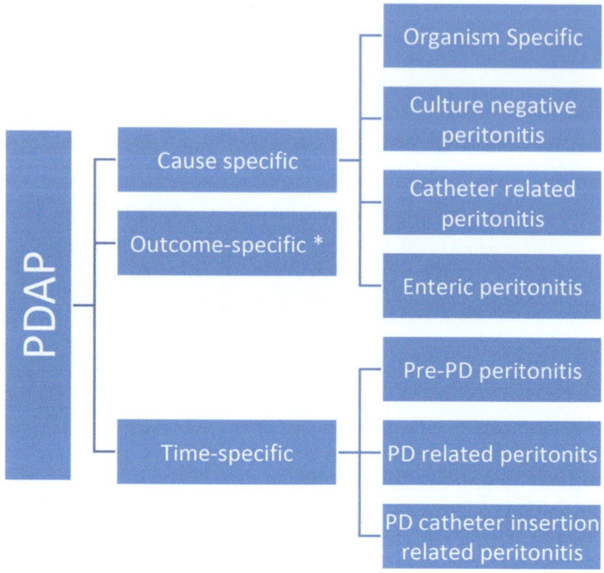

Fig. 3.2 Classification of peritoneal dialysis-associated peritonitis. *Organism-specific peritonitis is further classified as refractory, recurrent. Relapsing, repeat, peritonitis-associated catheter removal, peritonitis-associated hemodialysis transfer, peritonitis-associated death, and peritonitis-associated hospitalization [5]

3.5 Pathogenesis of Peritonitis

Peritonitis is caused by introduction of microorganisms while handling the sterile peritoneum. The microbes may enter during faulty catheter insertion techniques, mishandling during dialysis procedure or compromised host defenses.

The following are culprit sources leading to peritonitis in patients undergoing peritoneal dialysis:

1. Intraluminal contamination: It is a contamination with pathogenic skin bacteria because of faulty catheter insertion technique, mishandling of transfer set between exchanges (Fig. 3.3).
2. Periluminal contamination: A biofilm is a slimy film of microbes (bacteria/fungi) adhering the surface of the catheter. The catheter itself maybe a nidus for microbial growth or there maybe extension of exit site or tunnel infection (Fig. 3.3).
3. Transvesical migration: It is a microbial contamination from a bowel or rarely a vaginal leak.
4. Hematogenous dissemination: It may occur due to a remote source (e.g., dental procedures).
5. Compromised host defenses: The continuous presence of dialysis solution hampers the natural host defense mechanisms owing to high glucose concentration of dialysis fluids, low pH, and possible illusion of macrophage and cytokines [6].

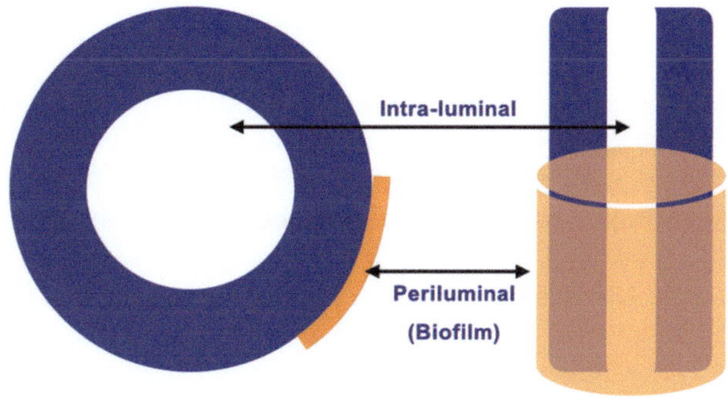

Fig. 3.3 Intraluminal and periluminal contamination

3.6 Risk Factors for PDAP

1. Invasive procedures like colonoscopy, cystoscopy, hysteroscopy, dental procedures
2. Nasal carriers of *Staphylococcus aureus*
3. Poor hygiene of the patient or caregiver and faulty technique while connecting/disconnecting transfer set
4. Others—constipation, hypoalbuminemia, gastrointestinal pathology, hypokalemia, smoking, and higher BMI [7]

3.7 Monitoring Patient with a PD Catheter

- The catheter insertion site is covered with a gauze dressing and adhesive tape to prevent the catheter from moving and to keep the area clean.
- Avoid repeated dressing unless soakage, as it disrupts the process of healing.
- The catheter insertion site and exit site along with the tunnel should be inspected for redness, tenderness, discoloration, or discharge and bleeding, on a daily basis. In order to prevent exit site leakage and infection, the exit site aperture should not be wide leading to gaping. The PD catheter should snuggly fit at the exit site. Suturing a gaped exit site incision acts like a nidus for infection and is best avoided.
- In and out flushes of catheter, to check patency in-between treatment sessions, are to be avoided, as they increase the chances of peritonitis.

Prevention of Peritonitis for USPD in Critically Ill (Box 1)

- Antibiotic/antifungal prophylaxis
- Tenckhoff catheter insertion
- Catheter insertion with strict aseptic precautions
- Y-transfer set (flush-before-fill technique)
- Topical antibiotic application for exit site care
- PD catheter immobilization
- Automated PD for ESPD
- Early detection and prompt treatment of exit site/tunnel infection

3.8 Practice Implications

Peritoneal dialysis-associated peritonitis is preventable, provided by strict adherence to the following:

1. Antibiotic prophylaxis at catheter insertion: a single dose of IV antibiotic (Vancomycin, Cephalosporin) has shown to decrease risk of early peritonitis.
   Administer systemic prophylactic antibiotics immediately prior to the following:
   (a) Catheter placement
   (b) Colonoscopy and invasive gynecological procedure
   (c) Wet contamination of the PD system to prevent peritonitis
       Antifungal prophylaxis (oral fluconazole 50 mg/day) [8] should be co-prescribed whenever PD patients receive an antibiotic course, regardless of the indication for that antibiotic course.
2. PD catheter design: systematic reviews (Strippoli et al., Hagen et al) [9, 10] compared the use of straight versus coiled catheters as well as straight versus swan neck catheters and found no significant difference in the risk of peritonitis, peritonitis rate, exit site/tunnel infection, and exit site/tunnel infection rate. The standard two-cuff Tenckhoff catheter insertion seems to be the best choice at present.
3. PD catheter insertion technique: method of PD catheter insertion should depend on local expertise at each unit. PD catheter insertion under local anesthesia, in the operating room, is preferred over bedside catheter insertion to maintain a sterile environment. The nephrologists inserted PD catheter seems to be the preferred option in many centers (Figs. 3.4 and 3.5).
4. PD connectology: The "flush before fill" technique has been an important advance in PD connectology, made possible by the advent of the double bag system, and is now a standard practice, responsible for a dramatic reduction in the incidence of PDAP, especially those due to gram-positive organisms. APD is the preferred modality for ESPD as it reduces the number of manual spikings needed to perform the treatment session and hence reduces chances of peritonitis, especially gram-positive cocci. Also, the work load on the ICU and PD staff is drastically reduced.
5. Microbiologic techniques: Usage of PD catheter tips to detect peritonitis is unreliable and to be avoided. Specialized microbiologic techniques such as Bactec technology (blood culture bottles with direct infusion of the PD fluid) for cultures, agents such Triton-X and Tween 80, and water lysis to lyse neutrophils and extrude internalized bacilli improve culture positivity. Microbiologic analysis of the entire PD bag is ideal (Fig. 3.6).
6. Exit site care: The most common causative organisms for exit site/tunnel infections are *Staphylococcus aureus* and *Pseudomonas aeruginosa.* ISPD guidelines recommend topical antibiotic application (Mupirocin) at catheter exit site. Exit

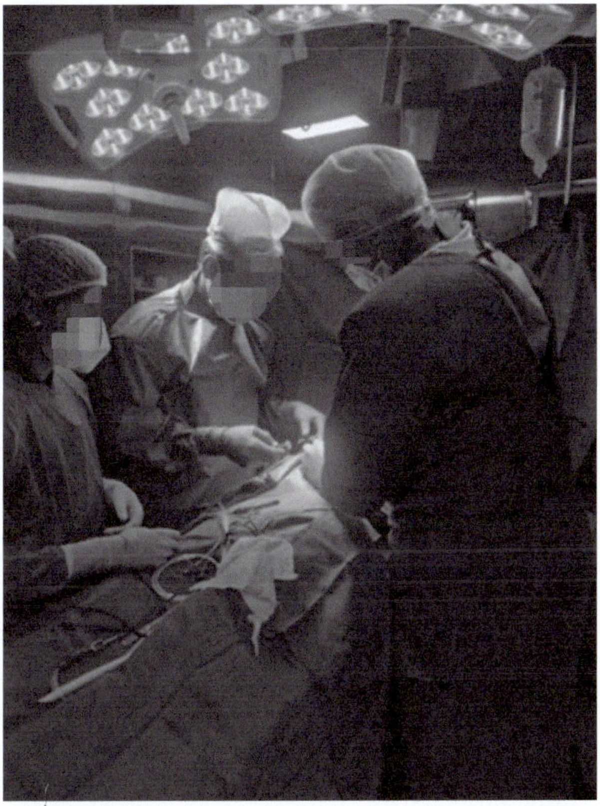

Fig. 3.4 PD catheter insertion by nephrologist team in the operating room

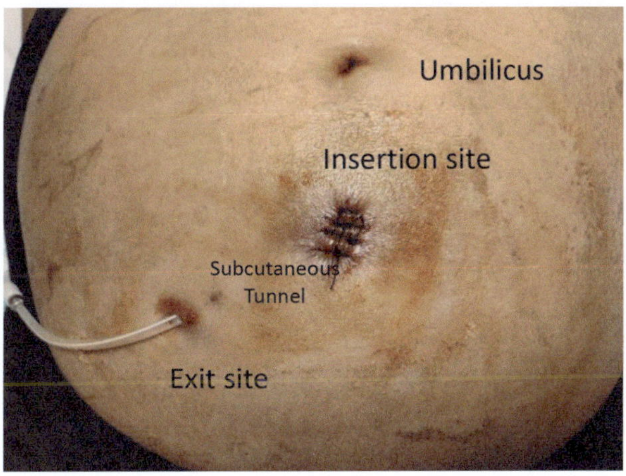

Fig. 3.5 Infraumbilical approach of catheter insertion with a subcutaneous tunnel

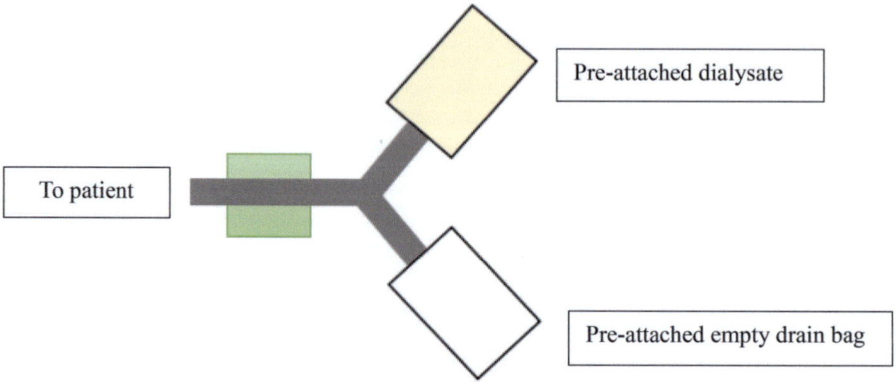

Fig. 3.6 Modified Y design of PD transfer set with pre-attached dialysis solution (yellow) and drain bag (clear) may lower the rates of peritonitis due to reduced handling

site or catheter tunnel infection must be treated promptly, for example, leaks or breaks in tubing proximal to the tubing clamp, leaks from dialysate bags, breach of aseptic technique, or touch contamination of the connection during a PD exchange.

7. PD catheter immobilization: Avoiding mechanical stress on the exit site and immobilization of PD catheter are advisable. Immobilizing the patient while PD treatment is ongoing, in the supine position with small volume exchanges, prevents exit site leakage. Prevention of exit site leakage is an important factor in reducing peritonitis, as this leads to wet contamination of the PD circuit.
8. Constipation must be avoided after catheter insertion to prevent transmigration of microbes. Treat hypokalemia and avoid or limit the use of histamine-2 receptor antagonists to prevent constipation.
9. Automated PD is advisable for emergent start PD in critically ill as dialysis can be delivered with minimal handling by the healthcare provider.

Take Home Message

- Emergent start peritoneal dialysis in the ICU is possible with the team work of nephrologist, PD nurses/care givers, ICU staff, pharmacist, and ancillary hospital support staff.
- Peritonitis among peritoneal dialysis patients is most often due to contamination with pathogenic skin bacteria, (*Staphylococcus epidermidis* and *Staphylococcus aureus*) while performing exchanges.

- Preventing peritonitis during emergent start PD is fundamental for successful treatment outcome in critically ill. After careful patient assessment, PD catheter insertion should be performed with strict aseptic precautions, by a skilled medical practitioner.
- The risk of peritonitis is lowered with the use of modified Y design of transfer set providing single-use disconnect system.
- Antibiotic/antifungal prophylaxis during PD catheter insertion and invasive intervention (colonoscopy, dental procedure) is mandatory.
- PD catheter insertion site, subcutaneous tunnel, and exit site should be inspected daily. The use of a topical antibiotic (Mupirocin) at the exit site prevents microbial contamination.
- Timely diagnosis of exit site/tunnel infections can reduce the risk of peritonitis (Fig. 3.7).

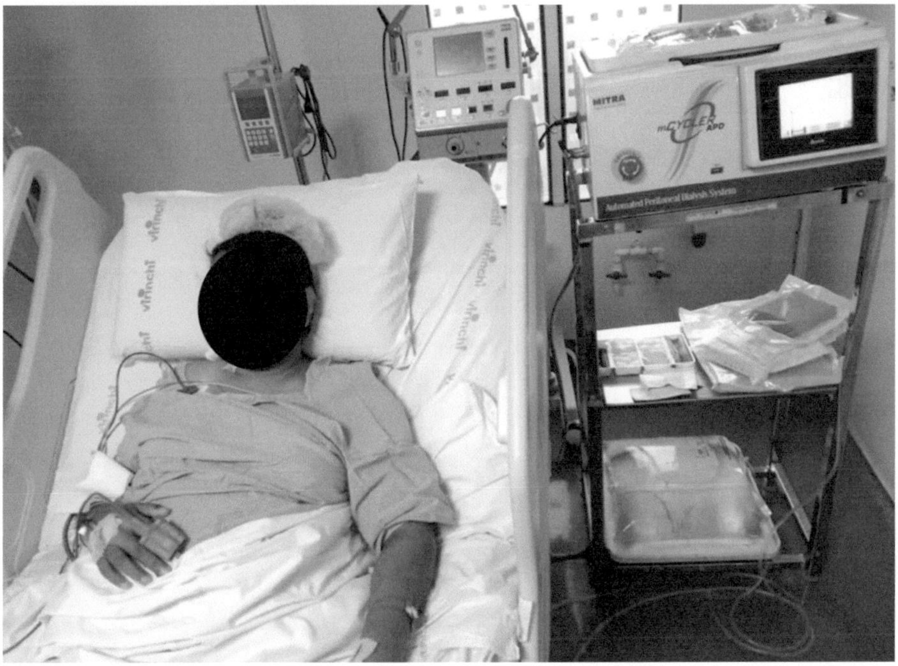

Fig. 3.7 Patient undergoing ESPD with APD in the ICU

References

1. Bowes E, Joslin J, Braide-Azikiwe DCB, Tulley C, Bramham K, Saha S, Jayawardene S, Shakoane B, Wilkins CJ, Hutchings S, Hopkins P, Lioudaki E, Shaw C, Cairns H, Sharpe CC. Acute peritoneal dialysis with percutaneous catheter insertion for COVID-19-associated acute kidney injury in intensive care: experience from a UK Tertiary center. Kidney Int Rep. 2021 Feb;6(2):265–71. https://doi.org/10.1016/j.ekir.2020.11.038.
2. Garg N, Kumar V, Sohal PM, Jain D, Jain A, VikasMakkar MS. Efficacy and outcome of intermittent peritoneal dialysis in patients with acute kidney injury: a single-center experience. Saudi J Kidney Dis Transpl. 2020. [cited 2022 Aug 26];31:423–30.
3. Htay H, Johnson DW, Craig JC, Teixeira-Pinto A, Hawley CM, Cho Y. Urgent-start peritoneal dialysis versus conventional-start peritoneal dialysis for people with chronic kidney disease. Cochrane Database Syst Rev. 2020;12:CD012913. https://doi.org/10.1002/14651858.CD012913.pub2.
4. Nayak KS, Subramanyam S, Pavvankumar N, Antony S. Emergent start peritoneal dialysis for end-stage renal disease: outcomes and advantages. Blood Purif. 2018;45:313–9. https://doi.org/10.1159/000486543.
5. Li PK-T, Chow KM, Cho Y, et al. ISPD peritonitis guideline recommendations: 2022 update on prevention and treatment. Perit Dial Int. 2022;42(2):110–53. https://doi.org/10.1177/08968608221080586.
6. Brulez HF, Verbrugh HA. First-line defense mechanisms in the peritoneal cavity during peritoneal dialysis. Perit Dial Int. 1995;15(7 Suppl):S24–33. discussion S33–4
7. Wu H, Huang R, Yi C, Wu J, Guo Q, Zhou Q, Yu X, Yang X. Risk factors for early-onset peritonitis in southern Chinese peritoneal dialysis patients. Perit Dial Int. 2016;36(6):640–6. https://doi.org/10.3747/pdi.2015.00203.
8. Prabhu MV, Sreepada V, et al. Prophylaxis against fungal peritonitis in CAPD–a single center experience with low-dose fluconazole. Ren Fail. 2010;32(7):802–5.
9. Strippoli GFM, Tong A, Johnson D, et al. Catheter type, placement and insertion techniques for preventing peritonitis in peritoneal dialysis patients. Cochrane Database Syst Rev. 2004;5:CD004680.
10. Hagen SM, Lafranca JA, Ijzermans JNM, et al. A systematic review and meta-analysis of the influence of peritoneal dialysis catheter type on complication rate and catheter survival. Kidney Int. 2014;85:920–32.

Peritonitis in CAPD: Microbiological Considerations in Diagnosis

4

Uma Sekar, Sheela Devi, and Archana Ashwin

4.1 Case Report

A 45 years old lady with CKD stage 5, a non-diabetic with idiopathic lung fibrosis, was on CAPD for 3 years. She had a swan neck TENCKHOFF double cuff catheter. She presented with symptoms of peritonitis Culture of the cloudy effluent grew *Pseudomonas aeruginosa*. There was no evidence of ESI (exit site infection). She was treated with intraperitoneal amikacin and meropenem and peritonitis resolved in a weeks' time. She received oral fluconazole also during the antibiotic therapy to prevent secondary fungal infections. The patient presented with features of recurrent peritonitis a day later and was again started on intraperitoneal amikacin and meropenem in recommended dosages. *Pseudomonas aeruginosa* was cultured again from the cloudy effluent. Oral fluconazole was continued. Dialysate fluid turned clear after 14 days of treatment. However, intermittent mild cloudiness of the peritoneal fluid was noted during the course of treatment. In view of this, the formation of a biofilm with in situ persistence of the organism was strongly suspected. The catheter was removed on completion of 14 days of therapy. The culture of catheter tip grew *Pseudomonas aeruginosa* in culture with the same susceptibility pattern as the previous effluent culture isolate. She was switched to intermittent hemodialysis. Since the patient had an umbilical hernia, a swan neck Georgi and

U. Sekar (✉)
Sri Ramachandra Medical College, Sri Ramachandra Institute of Higher Education and Research, Chennai, Tamil Nadu, India
e-mail: umasekar@sriramachandra.edu.in

S. Devi
Pondicherry Institute of Medical Sciences, Pondicherry, India

A. Ashwin
MGM Health Care, Chennai, Tamil Nadu, India

G. Abraham et al. (eds.), *Diagnosis and Management of Complications of Peritoneal Dialysis related Peritonitis*,
https://doi.org/10.1007/978-981-99-2275-8_4

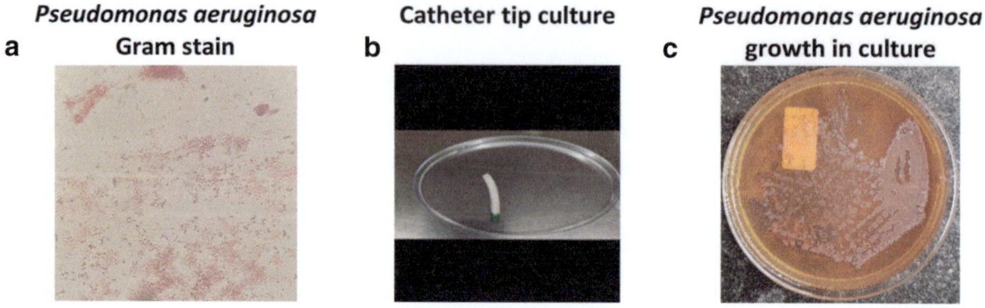

Fig. 4.1 (**a**) *Pseudomonas aeruginosa* gram stain (**b**) catheter tip culture (**c**) *Pseudomonas aeruginosa* growth in culture

Satish catheter was implanted a month later to continue PD. Peritoneal biopsy was done at the time of reimplantation. Gram's stain examination of peritoneal biopsy tissue was negative for presence of bacteria. A pericatheter collection of fluid was noted, and hence re-initiation of CAPD was postponed by a few days. The culture of this fluid was sterile (Fig. 4.1).

This is a case of relapsing *Pseudomonas aeruginosa* peritonitis in the absence of infection at the exit site but a possible tunnel infection requiring the removal of catheter with reimplantation at a later date.

4.2 Introduction

End stage renal disease requires renal replacement therapy as a lifesaving modality. Hemodialysis and peritoneal dialysis are the treatment options. However, the availability and access to a hemodialysis unit is a limiting factor for many patients in developing countries. Hence, peritoneal dialysis is a feasible modality in such patients. The two methods of peritoneal dialysis—the Continuous Ambulatory Peritoneal Dialysis (CAPD) and the Automated Peritoneal Dialysis (APD)—are both associated with peritonitis episodes. The latter is associated with reduced peritonitis rates, while relapse or recurrence rates are similar in both [1].

The occurrence of peritonitis is the single most limiting factor for the successful outcome of peritoneal dialysis and has largely hindered the acceptance of this modality. In 1976, Popovich first described this technique of CAPD as a treatment option for chronic renal failure. This initial technique has undergone several modifications to increase the convenience of the patient and to decrease the peritonitis risk and rates. Significantly, major modifications have been undertaken in the connector devices. [2].

The infection arises due to related processes or as a result of non-dialysis-related systemic or intra-abdominal causes. It has been documented that non-dialysis-related causes account for less than 6% of cases of peritonitis in CAPD patients. [3].

Methods for Reporting Peritonitis [4]

A. Number of infections that is caused by each organism over a specific period of time in relation to the number of dialysis years that the patient is at risk. It is usually expressed as rates and episodes per year.
B. Number of patients who are free of peritonitis over a time period. It is expressed as the percentage of patients.
C. Rate of peritonitis that occurs in each patient in a given program. It is expressed as the median peritonitis rates.

The International Society of Peritoneal Dialysis in 2016 considered a single episode of peritonitis every 2 years as a quality indicator to mark a successful PD therapy. [4] However, the treatment failure rates can be as high as 25%. [5, 6]. Infection has been identified as critically important, for the core outcomes in the SONG (Standardized Outcomes in Nephrology) initiative. [7].

Peritonitis resulting in structural changes in the peritoneal membrane is a major determinant contributing to substantial mortality in up to 8.6% of patients. [8] Significant morbidity, the loss of catheter, switching of the patient to hemodialysis, and ultimately damage to the peritoneal membrane that leads to temporary or permanent loss of ultrafiltration capabilities are other factors that have hampered the popularity of this modality worldwide. Even with early initiation of treatment, around 20% of all PD-related peritonitis episodes remain refractory to treatment. [9] Such severe, refractory, and persistent infections lead to more structural and functional alterations of the peritoneal membrane causing encapsulating peritoneal sclerosis. This is a rare but an irreversible sequela.

4.3 Pathogenesis

Unlike surgical peritonitis, in CAPD peritonitis, the infecting dose of organisms that is required to initiate a peritonitis episode is a minimal contaminating dose. Blood cultures are seldom positive unless a hematogenous route of infection is implicated. The distribution of etiological organisms is predominantly gram-positive, and most of them are skin colonizers or touch contaminants. However, in India and few developing countries, gram-negative bacteria are predominant pathogens. [10, 11].

4.4 Causative Agents of PD Peritonitis

Bacteria are the most frequent cause and originate mainly from contamination arising during a peritoneal dialysis session. Fungal infections are not as common as bacterial infections (only 3–6% of cases) but may occur subsequent to antibiotic use. [12, 13] Viruses are not usually implicated in peritonitis and parasites very rarely. Gram-positive pathogens are the most likely causative agents [14], but gram-negative pathogens are more commonly encountered in some centers. Organisms like *Pseudomonas aeruginosa* and fungi are associated with prolonged infection, worse outcomes, and, more importantly, PD failure. [9] Sequestration of the infection focus within the peritoneal cavity leads to abscess formation particularly when fecal flora or *Staphylococcus aureus* are involved. Even with optimal technique, 2 to 40% of cultures can be negative and yield no growth. [15, 16] (Table 4.1).

Surveillance cultures from abdominal site, nostrils, and hands of patients have been done in few PD units in an effort to ascertain if the organism causing the infection arose from the patient's own flora. Table 4.2 depicts the organisms isolated in 47 CAPD patients at different sites of surveillance sampling. 50 to 94% of the peritonitis isolates belonged to the same biotype isolated from their own flora. [2] Hence, patients are more at increased risk of acquiring the infection from their own resident flora rather than the environment or other persons. However, introduction of organisms (exogenous or endogenous) by touch contamination during the procedure is a major factor and has to be addressed with proper education of the patient and caregiver for the successful outcome of a PD program (Fig. 4.2).

Table 4.1 Etiological agents of peritonitis and their frequency of occurrence [2]

Coagulase negative staphylococci	30–40%
Staphylococcus aureus	20%
Streptococcus species	10–15%
Neisseria species	1–2%
Diphtheroid (Corynebacterium species)	1–2%
Escherichia coli	5–10%
Pseudomonas species	5–10%
Enterococcus species	3–6%
Klebsiella species	1–3%
Proteus species	3–6%
Acinetobacter species	2–5%
Anaerobic organisms	2–5%
Fungi (yeasts and molds)	2–10%
Mycobacteria	2–5%
Culture negative	0–30%

Table 4.2 Organisms cultured from body sites in patients on CAPD [2]

Organism	Hand (%)	Abdomen (%)	Nostril (%)	Total (%)
Coagulase negative Staphylococci	76	69	59	69
Staphylococcus aureus	3	4	7	13
Gram-negatives	3	4	8	15
Diphtheroid, yeast, etc.	15	18	20	53

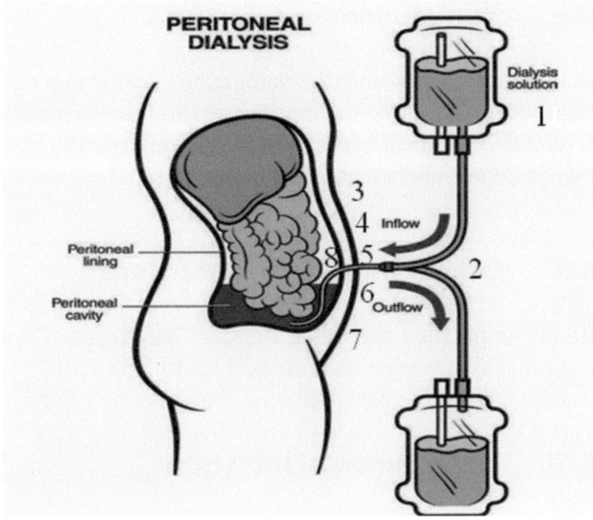

Fig. 4.2 External portals of entry

4.5 Intraluminal Infections

It occurs when the organisms gain access to the internal channels of the PD tubing through the internal surfaces or cracks in the tubing. Touching the tube with contaminated hands at the connector site during disconnection procedure also contributes to infection. Commercial dialysis fluids or the supplements like antibiotics added to the fluid connections are not generally considered to be portal or source of infection.

4.6 Periluminal Infections

Despite the cuffs in the catheter, an entirely sealed interface does not exist between the catheter and skin and subcutaneous tissue. Thus, penetration of organisms from around the catheter entry site is a possible portal. However, this route of entry is not considered a major one. One study found no difference in the peritonitis rate between patients who had occlusive dressing and patients who had no dressings and allowed to shower. [17] It is now known that an exit site or tunnel infection needs to be established before peritonitis sets in [18].

4.7 Transmural (Intestinal Infections)

A fecal leak is to be looked for if multiple bacteria of intestinal flora with or without anaerobes are isolated in culture. While bacteria do possess the ability to migrate through the intestinal wall, ischemic bowel disease and diverticulosis predispose to migration [19].

4.8 Hematogenous Infections

Remote infections with hematogenous seeding occur in some PD patients. The route of infection for tuberculous peritonitis is classically by this route. Similarly, *Streptococcus viridians* is thought to cause peritonitis following an upper respiratory infection via hematogenous spread [20].

4.9 Other Endogenous Infections

Rarely implicated are other sources like vagina. Candida peritonitis following a vaginal leak has been documented [21].

4.10 Environmental Infections

Environmental bacteria like Acinetobacter species and *Stenotrophomonas maltophilia* which cause peritonitis occasionally are thought to gain access to peritoneal cavity from water sources during bathing or swimming. Non-tuberculous mycobacterial infection can also be acquired by this route [22].

4.11 Biofilm

Biofilm on catheters is an unavoidable sequelae after catheter insertion. Their precise role in initiation of peritonitis remains uncertain though the microorganisms present in the biofilm matrix remain a constant source of infection due to the ease of access to the peritoneal cavity [23, 24].

Adherent biofilm microcolonies of bacteria on catheter surfaces obtain nutrition from dialysis effluents. Protected within the biofilm, the bacteria may undergo change in their genetic makeup or become more antibiotic resistant. Use of disconnect systems like twin bags, proper care of exit site with application of prophylactic antibiotics, surveillance cultures for colonization, and prophylactic antibiotics for carriers and use of "buried catheter" technique are some of the strategies that are directed towards prevention of biofilms [25]. Antibiotics like rifampicin and thrombolytic agents like streptokinase or urokinase have potency to disrupt of biofilms and facilitate the administered antibiotic to penetrate and act on the bacteria [26]. Alternatively, antibiotic "lock solutions" can be used in the catheter lumen which delivers microbicidal concentration of antibiotics at the site. [27] This has proven useful in prevention with recurrent peritonitis. Currently, studies are ongoing to evaluate the usefulness of various coatings on catheter lumen to prevent biofilm-related peritonitis.

4.12 Risk Factors for Infection

Patient-centered factors that increase the risk of infection include old age, smoking, obesity, diabetes, hypoalbuminemia, hypokalemia, lack of vitamin D supplement, inadequate training, prior exit site infection, and preceding peritonitis episodes [28].

4.13 Inflammatory Response in Peritonitis

When microorganisms enter the peritoneal cavity, an intense inflammatory response occurs with cellular proliferation and release of cytokines. The intrinsic fibrinolytic property of the peritoneal membrane is compromised during inflammation resulting in delayed breakdown of fibrin and formation of fibrin strands in the cavity. Fibronectin is thus seen in increased concentrations in the peritoneal fluid during episodes of peritonitis. Once invasion of organism occurs, there is a heightened cellular response resulting in an influx of polymorphonuclear leucocytes [29]. The cellular response may be varied with predominant lymphocytes or eosinophils in accordance with the pathogenic process. [30].

Cellular response—A cloudy effluent is more frequently caused by increase in the number of cells of any type with or without the presence of infection. Among patients with cloudy effluent, the predominant cell type is identified by cellular analysis of the fluid either by manual examination and counting of cell types by microscopy or by automated cell counters which evaluate and determine the cell count and type within a very short time span.

Cellular types encountered in cloudy effluent with or without peritonitis:

- Atypical cells—Lymphoma or other malignancy
- Neutrophils—In addition to bacterial infection, exposure to certain drugs (amphotericin, vancomycin) [31], renal cell carcinoma [32], pancreatitis and other retroperitoneal disease, leukemia, intra-abdominal disease, lymphoma [33], and icodextrin dialysate [34]
- Eosinophils—In addition to bacterial infection, fungal and viral infections, allergic reactions, drug effects (such as vancomycin), early after catheter placement as a result of CO_2 insufflation during laparoscopy, following peritonitis, icodextrin dialysate, intraperitoneal vancomycin [35]
- Monocytes—In addition to bacterial infection, mycobacterial infection and icodextrin dialysate
- Erythrocytes—Trauma during placement of the dialysis catheter and gynecologic disorders, ovulation, or menses. Bloody dialysate can occasionally occur in routine infectious peritonitis [36]

4.14 Peritonitis in PD: Definitions

Primary peritonitis: refers to the focus of infection confined to the peritoneal cavity.

Secondary peritonitis: is the resultant peritonitis following infection in the gastrointestinal tract or very rarely due to a hematogenous seeding of the peritoneum ensuing a bacteremia episode. Examples of gastrointestinal infections and conditions that may precede a CAPD peritonitis include cholecystitis, appendicitis, diverticulitis, severe persistent constipation, bowel ischemia, and perforation due to any underlying pathology or a strangulated hernia. Bacteremia episodes that result in secondary peritonitis include endoscopic procedures of the gastrointestinal tract and dental procedures. Seeding may also occur from the vagina in females. The prognosis in secondary peritonitis is less favorable when compared to primary peritonitis.

Relapsing peritonitis
Is defined as an episode that occurs within 4 weeks of completion of therapy of a prior episode with the same organism (may be culture negative in the second episode).

Recurrent peritonitis
Is defined as an episode that occurs within 4 weeks of completion of therapy of a prior episode but with a different organism.

Repeat peritonitis
Is defined as an episode that occurs >4 weeks after completion of therapy of a prior episode with the same organism or 5 weeks after the last dose of antibiotic if the patient was treated with a long-acting agent such as vancomycin.

Refractory peritonitis
Failure of the effluent to clear after 5 days of therapy with appropriate antibiotics.

Catheter-related peritonitis
Occurs in conjunction with an exit site or tunnel infection with the same organism.

Role of Microbial virulence factors in pathogenicity
The microbial virulence factors contribute to pathogenicity and severity of infection. [37] They include

A. Colonization potential and adherence to epithelial cells or catheter surfaces to form biofilms
B. Evasion of host defense by intracellular sequestration
C. Rate of multiplication of the microbe
D. Host tissue damage caused

Microorganisms like *Staphylococcus aureus* and fungi like candida produce abundant extracellular slime which enhances their colonization potential. The formation of biofilm protects them from host defense and allows their survival in microcolonies within the film. Such persistence of organisms within the biofilm contributes to recurrence of infection. Gram-negatives like *Pseudomonas aeruginosa* and few Enterobacteriaceae also possess colonization potential by means of fimbria and certain cell wall components.

Staphylococci are among one of the hardiest bacteria and can survive in many non-physiological environmental conditions. They equally colonize the immunocompetent and compromised. At least 30% of any population will be permanent and another 30% intermittent carriers of staphylococci. Generally, patients transfer the organism from the anterior nares to the catheter site skin through their hands. Skin and hand disinfection therefore are of paramount importance. Their indolence and predilection to harbor multiple antimicrobial resistance genes make them a formidable pathogen. Decolonization measures may not permanently get rid of these organisms though the bioburden may be reduced at the colonized sites. The methicillin-resistant biotype of staphylococcus (MRSA and MR Coagulase negative Staphylococci) is resistant to all beta lactam and beta lactam inhibitor combination of antibiotics and thus poses a therapeutic challenge.

Pseudomonas is a cosmopolitan gram-negative bacillus predominantly deemed as an environmental bacterium. It can survive with minimum nutrients under extreme environmental conditions. It colonizes the moist wet surfaces of the human body, and such colonization precedes invasive infection. This species is known to acquire resistance to multiple drugs and also to commonly used disinfectants.

Candida is a part of the resident flora of humans in the human gastrointestinal tract and skin. Most infections originate endogenously. Prolonged antibiotic therapy for bacterial peritonitis predisposes to Candida overgrowth and peritonitis. [38] An ascending infection from vagina in women with intra uterine contraceptive device has been documented. [39] Deficiency of certain complement components combined with the deficiency of immunoglobulins and hyperglycemic environment favors candida multiplication and infection. [40]. The emergence of Candida species that are intrinsically resistant or have reduced susceptibility to frontline antifungal drugs is a cause for concern.

Enterobacteriaceae include *Escherichia coli, Klebsiella pneumoniae*, and a host of other species form normal flora of the gastrointestinal tract. Among gram-negatives, they are the prime contributors for infection. In the immunosuppressed and hospitalized, they colonize the skin and upper respiratory tract. Resistance to multiple antibiotics and the ability to acquire resistance are a notable feature of this group of bacteria. Resistance to all cephalosporins and carbapenems is becoming commonplace in this group of bacteria. Infections with gram-negative bacteria resistant to multiple antibiotics is an emerging concern in many countries today. [41].

Enterococcus species also forms part of the normal gastrointestinal flora. Among the various species, *Enterococcus faecium* is known for its propensity to acquire vancomycin resistance.

Acinetobacter and *Stenotrophomonas* species are typical examples of environmental bacteria and considered opportunistic pathogens in a variety of clinical settings. Placement of in dwelling devices serves as a platform through which these bacteria gain access and acquire pathogenicity.

4.15 Mycobacterium Species and Tuberculous Peritonitis

Tuberculosis is a prime global health problem and is endemic in many countries. The pathogenesis of peritoneal tuberculosis in patients undergoing CAPD remains unclear. Patients with end-stage renal disease (ESRD) have relative deficiency of cell-mediated immunity which is required to prevent active tuberculosis. Patients with ESRD have 5–15 times higher susceptibility for developing active tuberculosis than the general population [42]. Additionally, extrapulmonary tuberculosis is also more common. Diabetes mellitus and local immunodeficiency in the peritoneal cavity are known risk factors for tuberculosis. The attributable mortality due to peritoneal tuberculosis in patients undergoing CAPD is estimated to be 15%. Delay in diagnosis and treatment attributes to mortality. Non-tuberculous mycobacteria, e.g., *Mycobacterium fortuitum* and *Mycobacterium chelonei*, are environmental organisms. Many of them are likely to be more resistant to first-line antituberculosis drugs [43]. Treatment options vary for non-tuberculous mycobacteria. Once a mycobacteria is isolated in culture, it is imperative for the laboratory to identify the species because of the varied treatment protocols. Abraham et al. conducted a prospective study of 155 patients who were initiated on CAPD [44]. In their cohort, four patients developed tuberculous peritonitis. These patients had been on PD for a duration of 2–84 months. The authors concluded that, although TB peritonitis constituted a mere 1–2% of all peritonitis episodes, in culture negative peritonitis, a high index of suspicion of TB is required. The various options for diagnosis include Ziehl–Nielsen-stained smear, Auramine O fluorescence-based microscopy, culture by conventional or automated methods, and PCR [44].

Once a diagnosis of peritonitis is made, empirical treatment is initiated after obtaining the effluent for culture. After obtaining the culture results, treatment can be tailored or targeted in order to preserve the function of the peritoneal membrane. The time interval between the onset of peritonitis and treatment is an independent risk factor for PD failure and increases by 6.8% for every hour of delay in the intuition of antibiotics [45]. Antibiotics are administered optimally by the intraperitoneal route because a high concentration is achieved in the peritoneum. In addition, an intravenous access can be avoided, and administration can be continued at home by trained personnel [45].

4.16 Diagnosis of Peritonitis

The presenting symptoms of peritonitis vary in patient populations. Abdominal pain and cloudy effluent remain the most common symptom and sign. The following are the findings associated with the development of peritonitis [46].

- Abdominal pain—79 to 88%
- Fever (greater than 37.5 °C)—29 to 53%

- Nausea or vomiting—31 to 51%
- Cloudy effluent—84%
- Hypotension—18%
- Chills—20 to 30%
- Redness or swelling at the catheter exit site.
- Loss of appetite, fatigue

Onset of pain and the appearance of cloudy fluid may not occur at the same time. Some patients, present with pain with clear dialysate fluid. The fluid turns cloudy a day later or after the next exchange [47].

The severity of abdominal pain varies with the causative organism too. The more virulent a pathogen, the more likely is the severity of symptoms and less favorable the treatment outcomes. [8, 48].

Physical examination reveals abdominal tenderness and rebound tenderness, though guarding is rarely present. A localized abdominal pain should raise suspicion of underlying surgical pathology since precise localization of pain or tenderness is observed in patients with secondary peritonitis due to specific underlying pathology. Occasionally, systemic signs of sepsis, including hypotension, may be present. Patients with secondary peritonitis may also have systemic manifestations of sepsis [49].

Among patients who are febrile or appear septic, additional tests to determine the source of infection is warranted. This may include obtaining blood cultures and tests considered as markers of sepsis. Radiographic studies do not have additional value and hence not performed as part of routine work up. However, computed tomography (CT) of the abdomen can be of value in some patients for detecting loculated fluid collections or abscess, thickening of the small-bowel wall or adhesions, and exclusion of other causes of intra-abdominal sepsis [50]. The culture of multiple enteric organisms generally points to a secondary peritonitis from a gastrointestinal source, including the possibility of a perforated viscus. For such patients, imaging and additional analysis of serum and peritoneal fluid are required. CT scan can be performed for patients with infection due to multiple enteric organisms, especially in those who fail to respond to appropriate antimicrobial treatment clinically or biochemically; patients with hypotension or those with hemodynamic instability; patients with concurrent bacteremia; and patients with localized pain or increased severity of symptoms suggestive of a secondary pathology or abnormal blood test results such as elevated lipase, bilirubin, or transaminase enzyme levels [51].. Mild elevation in serum lactate level during episodes of peritonitis can be the due of delayed metabolism of the lactate buffer used in the PD solutions rather than tissue hypoperfusion or bowel ischemia [52].

History of recent contamination, accidental disconnection, endoscopic or gynecologic procedure, constipation, or diarrhea should be sought from every patient. Details of previous episodes of peritonitis or exit site infection should also be elicited. Inspection of the catheter tunnel and exit site should be performed for evidence of discharge. The discharge fluid must be subjected to culture [53].

4.17 Confirmed Diagnosis of Peritonitis

Peritonitis is confirmed by a positive culture in 80–95% of cases provided the appropriate culture technique is followed [54].

In instances where the culture of the dialysate remains negative in spite of clinical signs and symptoms, a diagnosis of peritonitis may still be made if two or more of the following criteria are present [4, 18].

- Suggestive clinical features (abdominal pain or cloudy effluent)
- Raised white cell count in the peritoneal fluid greater than 100 cells/mm^3 (or 0.1 × 10^9/L after dwell time of at least 2 h). Relative increase in neutrophil count of greater than 50%
- Positive effluent culture
- If the patient has an infectious cause of peritonitis, but the culture is consistently negative, it may be due to one or more of the following reasons:
- The culture is obtained early in the course, before the microorganism load or numbers are not high enough for isolation in vitro.
- Incorrect microbiologic culture technique, most common being collection of inadequate volume of effluent for sampling [55].
- Antibiotics administered for other reasons before or during the time of sampling and not neutralized during the process of culture [56]. Such cultures require prolonged incubation for growth to occur and neutralization of antibiotics in vitro.
- Intermittent release of the organisms into the peritoneal cavity an intracellular or fastidious organisms [57]. This includes mycobacteria and fungi which need prolonged incubation and specific culture media to support growth.
- Endotoxin released by the sequestrated organism in the absence of free viable bacteria in the fluid also elicits an intense inflammatory response without a positive culture [58].

Cloudy peritoneal effluent—Multiple conditions result in a cloudy effluent. The cause can be ascertained upon analysis of the effluent.

Patients on PD presenting with a cloudy effluent should be presumed to have peritonitis and treated until the diagnosis is excluded. It is mandatory to test the effluent for cell count, differential count, gram stain, and culture.

Though a cloudy effluent generally points to an infectious peritonitis, there could be other causes such as enumerated below. A dialysate that is cloudy due to an infectious process has certain attributes like low pH (5.5 to 6), high osmolarity, low immunoglobulins, and demonstrable reduction in the phagocytic activity of the neutrophils.

Conditions that cause cloudy effluent may be classified according to the attributing substance – noncellular or cellular. The cellular types have been already discussed.

Noncellular causes for cloudy effluent are as follows [59]

- Excessive fibrin production. This may occur at initiation of peritoneal dialysis and occasionally after peritonitis. Excessive fibrin results in presence of filaments and sometimes a clot in the dialysis fluid.
- Effluent was obtained after a prolonged period of peritoneal rest (i.e., no peritoneal dialysis or "dry" abdomen).
- A triglyceride or lipid leakage in the cavity (chylous ascites). This arises from obstruction of the lymphatics due to a malignant focus like lymphoma, acute pancreatitis, and superior vena cava syndrome. Rarely, it can occur due to the usage of dihydropyridine calcium channel blockers.
- Severe constipation and a prolonged dwell time.

Hence, abdominal pain and cloudy effluent are not always due to peritonitis. Certain conditions including ischemic colitis, pancreatitis, pyelonephritis, ruptured ovarian or kidney cyst, transplant kidney rejection, *Clostridium* difficile infection, and strangulated/incarcerated hernia can also produce similar signs and symptoms.

Elevated eosinophilic count of 10–30% occurs in eosinophilic peritonitis. This condition typically occurs in the first few weeks of PD initiation and is presumably due to an allergic reaction to the PD solution, plasticizers, tubing, air, vancomycin, streptokinase, or the PD catheter itself. There is concomitant elevation of eosinophils in the peripheral blood count. This condition resolves spontaneously within a few months. Low-dose corticosteroid therapy or antihistamines can be helpful in clearing the cloudiness of the effluent. [60].

Cytology and flow cytometry can be helpful in persistent sterile cloudy effluent especially to rule out malignant and other type of cells in the dialysate. [61].

When there is a milky white effluent, it is desirable to check the triglyceride levels to rule out chylous effluent which is typically acellular but rich in triglycerides (higher dialysate levels compared with serum). Normally serum triglyceride level is lower than the dialysate triglyceride levels. The levels may vary as per the dietary fat consumption.

Approximately 10% of peritoneal dialysis patients with bacterial peritonitis have dialysate white cell counts below 100/mm^3. A low white cell count with peritonitis is commonly due to a short dwell time. A poor host immune response can also contribute to delayed or diminished increase in the peritoneal fluid white cell count [62].

4.18 Peritoneal Fluid Culture

Peritoneal fluid culture is positive in approximately 80 to 95% of peritonitis cases provided that proper culture technique is followed. Culture by whatever method adopted remains the standard investigation to confirm peritonitis.

The collection, transport, and processing of the sample are crucial and should be standardized in all laboratories serving patients on PD. The yield in culture improves with standardized improved techniques. The first cloudy bag (Fig. 4.3) before the initiation of antibiotic treatment is the optimal sample for the laboratory. Patients can be instructed to bring the first cloudy bag in the event of them coming to the PD center from their homes. They can be instructed to refrigerate the bag in case of delay in transport to the laboratory (4° to 8°C).

It is optimal to submit the entire bag containing the cloudy effluent to the laboratory. The bag should be labeled properly with details of patient and date/time of collection (Fig. 4.4). Other details including information about previous episodes of peritonitis and antibiotic administration if any during/before the collection should be provided to laboratory for appropriate diagnostic work up. The laboratory personnel can visually inspect the fluid and draw the required quantity from the bag following strict aseptic precautions. This helps to avoid external contamination during the process and prevents the contaminants growing in culture. Since any contaminating bacteria can be the pathogen as well, care should be taken by the laboratory personnel to prevent external contamination during the process of culture inoculation.

Fig. 4.3 Cloudy bag

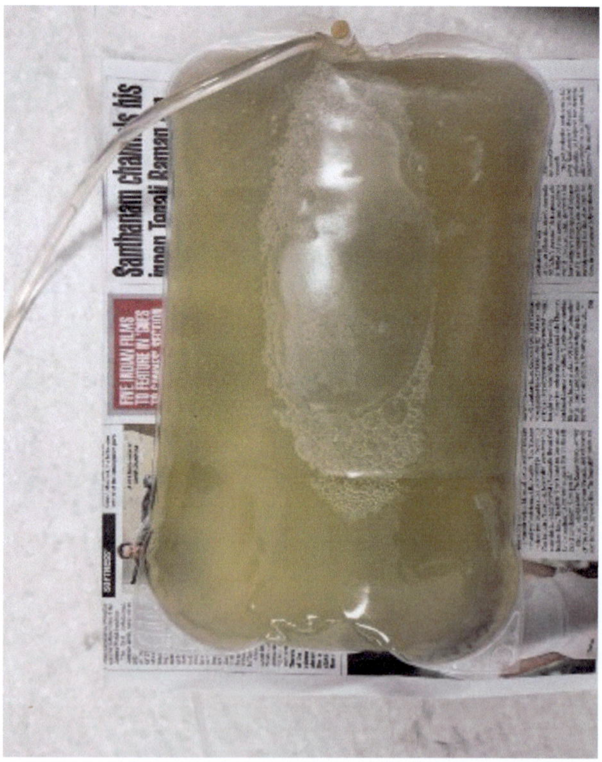

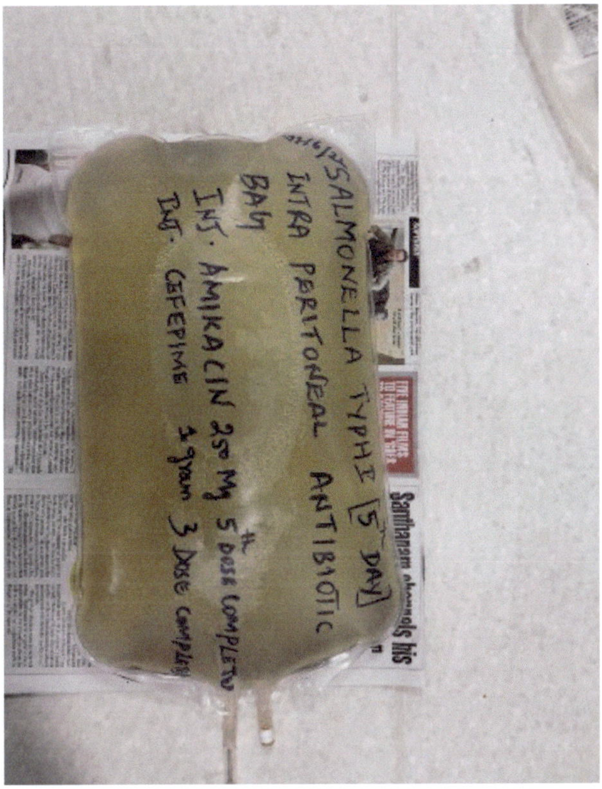

Fig. 4.4 Bag labeling

The bag should be submitted to the laboratory as early as is possible preferably within 6 h of collection. Multiplication and metabolic activity of bacteria within the fluid releases acidic residues which can adversely affect the yield of bacteria in culture. Further, the viability of bacteria is lost during a prolonged transport time. In case of anticipated delay, the bag can be refrigerated at 4–8 °C without subjecting to freeze. Direct bedside inoculation of 5 to 10 mL of effluent into 2 (aerobic and anaerobic) blood-culture bottles is also recommended provided these are available on site.

With well-equipped laboratory and trained microbiology personnel, the rate of culture-negative peritonitis can be substantially reduced. Once the sample is received in the laboratory, it is subjected to biochemical analysis, cell count/typing, and microbiological investigations. The laboratory personnel can visualize the fluid to look for clots, flakes, or fibrin strands and then draw the sample from the bag. It is worthwhile to include the fibrin strands if any while drawing the sample. The fibrin strands harbor the trapped bacteria from the fluid. Concentrating the effluent and subsequent washing of the effluent before culture inoculation free these entrapped bacteria thus improving the chances of their recovery in culture.

When patients present to the emergency department, the optimal culture technique is often not adopted resulting in negative cultures. [63] Conversely, when they present to a PD unit, the chance of recovery and identification is increased because of sensitization to and awareness of the appropriate techniques among the staff of a PD unit.

The organisms that are cultured from peritoneal fluid differ in peritoneal dialysis-related and secondary peritonitis. In the former, gram-positive organisms (usually coagulase-negative *Staphylococcus* species) are the most common, whereas enteric organisms (such as *Bacteroides*) or culture of multiple organisms are often observed in secondary peritonitis [64, 65]. In the absence of fever or signs of sepsis, blood cultures are generally negative among patients with both PD-related and secondary peritonitis. Most studies have shown that coagulase-negative staphylococci are the predominant organisms and account for 27.5 to 60% of all positive cultures followed by *Staphylococcus aureus* and *Streptococcus* including *Enterococci* (10 to 20% each). Enterobacteriaceae (10 to 20%), non-fermenting gram-negative bacteria including *Pseudomonas aeruginosa* (5–15%), gram-positive rods (2–5%), mixed organisms, fungi (including algae), mycobacteria, and anaerobes account for the other type of infections (Table 4.3).

Table 4.3 depicts the possible causes of peritonitis in relation to the etiological agent and the containment measures to be adopted in each setting [50]

Organism	Possible cause	Recommended action
Coagulase-negative staphylococcal species and *Staphylococcus aureus*	Breach in sterile technique during connection and coexisting exit site infection	Patient education; care and treatment of exit site infection
Streptococcus	Dental procedures; GI flora translocation	Prophylaxis for dental and endoscopic procedures; treatment of dental and periodontal disease
Enteric organisms (gram-negative rods and anaerobes)	Intra-abdominal pathology; severe constipation/GI procedures	Avoid constipation; antibiotic prophylaxis for endoscopic procedures; CT scan to rule out GI leak and perforation
Fungus	Prior antibiotic therapy/ immunocompromised state	Antifungal prophylaxis during prolonged antibiotic therapy
Pseudomonas aeruginosa	Exit site and tunnel infection	Exit site and catheter care
Pasteurella species	Domestic pets, mainly cats	Patient education on avoiding contact with pets during exchanges and exit site care
Culture negative	Prior antibiotic therapy; suboptimal culturing techniques	Review culturing methods and specimen handling; culture for unusual/fastidious organisms (i.e., TB)

4.19 Microbiologic Culture Technique

An optimal technique for culturing peritoneal fluid among continuous ambulatory peritoneal dialysis (CAPD) and automated peritoneal dialysis (APD) patients is the combination of sediment culturing from 50 mL effluent and bedside inoculation of 3 to 5 mL of effluent dialysate in each of two blood culture bottles [8]. Centrifugation of at least 50 mL of PD fluid and resuspending the sediment are the standard culture technique. As applicable to blood cultures, the more the volume of fluid sampled, the more the chances of recovery of the pathogen in culture [66].

For sediment culturing, at least 50 mL of dialysate fluid is centrifuged at 3000 g (i.e., relative centrifugal force) for 15 min and the supernatant is decanted off. The sediment is resuspended in 3 to 5 mL of sterile normal saline or a buffer. The sediment thus suspended can be vortexed for 1 to 2 min to dislodge the fibrin and the glucose overlay or coating on bacteria and to facilitate their growth in culture. It can be centrifuged again to obtain the final sediment for culture [67].

The final sediment obtained is inoculated on solid culture medium—McConkey agar, 5% sheep blood agar, chocolate agar, and into standard blood culture bottles (Aerobic and anaerobic). The culture plates are incubated at 37 °C and inspected for growth every day. Prolonged incubation is required for fastidious organisms and in cases where antibiotics have been administered to the patient before the sample collection. If fungus is implicated, use of fungus-specific medium like Sabouraud's Dextrose agar with or without bacteria inhibiting antibiotics incorporated in the media is used which permits the growth of fungus with relative inhibition of bacteria. Some molds require incubation at room temperatures. (22° to 28 °C).

The use of automated culture systems like BacT Alert /BACTEC increases the sensitivity of culture recovery and decreases the turnaround time due to continuous monitoring for evidence of growth and flagging of positive bottles. They also avoid the need to manually subculture at defined intervals, thus minimizing contamination during the process. Continuous monitoring for growth is possible at all times of the day. BacT/AlerT fastidious antimicrobial neutralization (FAN) plus blood culture bottles can be used. FANPlus is a resin-based media containing antibiotic-binding polymeric beads in place of charcoal-based antimicrobial neutralization. [56].

Use of lysis centrifugation method wherein the peritoneal fluid is treated with a solution of saponin and sodium polyanetholesulfonate (SPS) which break down the polymorphonuclear leucocytes and release the intracellular bacteria offers advantage in terms of rapid time to positivity and earlier identification of the pathogen by gram's stain and/or culture [68].

The international society of peritoneal dialysis (ISPD) guidelines recommend use of blood culture bottles for culture of the effluents. In most cases (75%), identification of the causative organism is known in about 72 h. Subculture on media with aerobic and/or microaerophilic incubation for 3 to 4 days may help identify slow-growing fastidious bacteria and yeasts that are undetectable by some automated culturing systems. Once the organism is grown in culture identification of the species can be obtained early by use of automated identification systems such as Vitek 2 or by MALDITOF (matrix-assisted laser desorption/ionization-time of flight (MALDI-TOF) mass spectrometry. Rapid and accurate identification of even rare species of bacteria, mycobacteria, and certain fungal pathogens can be obtained in a well-equipped clinical microbiology laboratory [69, 70]. For all organisms that are cultured, antimicrobial susceptibility testing is mandatory since susceptibilities are variable in each species of bacteria, acquired resistance is increasingly common, and some species are inherently resistant to certain classes of antibiotics.

If mycobacteria are suspected, the sample after the initial process should be inoculated into mycobacteria-specific medium—MGIT (mycobacteria growth indicator tube) MB Bac-T which contains enriched medium for growth and is an automated system which flags the positive growth in culture. They may also be inoculated into conventional solid medium like Lowenstein-Jensen agar, but this requires prolonged incubation. Once growth occurs, species identification and susceptibility testing are mandatory in view of the increased resistance encountered to antituberculosis drugs. There are several molecular methods now available for the work up of a tuberculous etiology including the molecular assays. [71].

4.20 Initial Smear Examination

Gram's Stain A carefully examined gram's stain smear establishes the presence of the microorganism only in about 20% to 30% of the cases but can be higher with a more experienced microbiologist. [72] This may not be a sufficiently sensitive test to initiate early directed therapy. Nevertheless, presumptive therapy can be started if positive and later modified as per culture and susceptibility report. Gram's stain allows the identification of yeasts also [72].

Zeihl Neilson Stain Smear is carefully examined for the presence of acid-fast bacilli. At least 100 oil immersion fields have to be examined microscopically. However, the sensitivity is low, and seldom are the mycobacteria visualzed in the smear [73].

4.21 Other Stains

Auramine-O Can be used to increase the sensitivity of the smear examination for mycobacteria. It is a fluorescent staining technique, and examination is done with the high-power objective of the microscope.

Calcofluor white Is also a fluorescent staining technique to examine for fungal elements in the fluid.

Wet mount preparation with 10% potassium hydroxide Fungal elements if present are best examined in 10% KOH wet mounts. Their morphology is noted to ascertain the presence of yeast cells or filamentous hyphal cells with the characteristic branching features and presence or absence of septa within the filaments to presumptively identify the class of fungi. Yeasts appear as round to oval bodies with or without budding and pseudohyphae in case of *Candida albicans*.

To enhance the recovery of peritoneal organisms among automated peritoneal dialysis (APD) patients who do not use a daytime exchange, it is optimal to infuse 1 liter of dialysate and allow it to dwell for a minimum of 2 h; the dialysate is then drained and examined for turbidity and sent for cell count and cell differential and culture [74].

The effluent can be sent to the laboratory more than once during the course of treatment. It is recommended to repeat the cultures every 3 days to ensure the progress and proper management [75]. Cell counts with differential counts can be estimated daily as a guide to therapy. If cultures are persistently positive and the cell counts show a rising trend, other focus of infection such as a remote focus, exit site, or tunnel infections has to be sought and treatment protocols revisited.

Clearing of the fluid (such that a newsprint if held behind the bag can be read through the bag), reduction in the cellular count, and negative cultures even after 1 week of incubation are pointers to the recovery and successful treatment of peritonitis (Fig. 4.5).

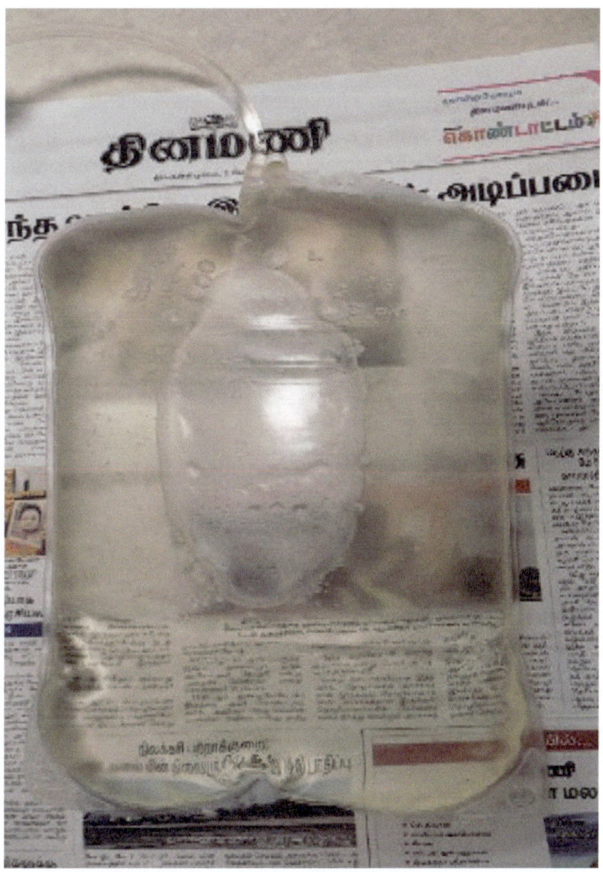

Fig. 4.5 Clear fluid after therapy

4.22 Microbiological Investigations in Exit Site and Tunnel Infections

Twardowski and Prowant's exit site classification system [76]

	Score		
Criteria	0 point	1 point	2 points
Swelling	No	Exit only (< 0.5 cm)	Including part of or entire tunnel
Crust	No	<0.5 cm	>0.5 cm
Redness	No	<0.5 cm	>0.5 cm
Pain on pressure	No	Slight	Severe
Secretion	No	Serous	Purulent

A score of 2 and above is indicative of infection. An equivocal score may indicate a developing peritonitis and hence needs monitoring and follow-up. [77]. Purulent secretion even in the absence of other signs is a positive indication of exit site infection.

Swabs are collected from the exit site if there are signs of infection. To avoid skin contaminants growing in swab culture, the area is first cleaned with sterile saline and allowed to dry for some time. Any fluid/pus coming out of the site is expressed, and swabs are applied to the fluid carefully avoiding the adjacent skin surface. The swabs are transported to the laboratory without delay. Ideally two swabs can be obtained—one used for smear study and the other subjected to culture.

It is prudent to send the catheter also for culture if removed. The inner tip of the catheter is cultured on suitable solid media by roll plate technique. Use of liquid enrichment media or broth is however not recommended. In case of long-standing catheters, with a possible biofilm, the catheter can be cut open with sterile precautions, inner surface of catheter with the biofilm layer scraped off gently, and the scrapings used for culture.

4.23 Recent Advances in the Diagnostic Methods for PD-Related Peritonitis [78]

4.23.1 Point of Care Testing

Leukocyte esterase are enzymes produced by activated white cells and serve as a marker of inflammation. The sensitivity, specificity, positive predictive value, and negative predictive value for cases based on clinical signs are determined to be 76.2%, 97.2%, 80%, and 96.6%, respectively, and the values as compared to the peritoneal cell counts have been determined as 90.5%, 98.6%, 95%, and 98.6%, respectively [79]. When compared to the cell count for its positive predictive value, it is estimated to be 74.1% vs 95% for cell count which undermines its use as an effective screening test. However, the test can be used in situations where the laboratory facilities are not readily available and the patient or caregiver can themselves screen the fluid for ruling out an infectious etiology.

Proinflammatory cytokines Are potential markers for diagnosing peritonitis. These are produced by activated cells during the inflammatory response. There are commercial test kits available as lateral flow assays which offer reports within hours [80].

A. Interleukin 6 (IL-6)
B. Cyclooxygenase-2 (COX-2)
C. Matrix metalloproteinase (MMP)-8

Studies have determined a significant correlation between number of episodes of peritonitis and IL-6 and COX-2 levels after 1 year of a peritonitis episode. MMP-8 is produced by activated neutrophils during acute inflammation. MMP-8 has been detected in the PD effluent of polymicrobial peritonitis [81]. A cut-off value that provides a good positive predictive value is yet not completely known. This restricts their use as a routine screening tool. However, IL-6 and MMP-8, in the peritoneal dialysate using a lateral flow assay device, has a high negative predictive value of 98.3% and positive predictive values of 83.7% with a high sensitivity and specificity of 97.6% and 87.7%, respectively. [81]. All the above markers if found negative reasonably rule out an infectious process, thus minimizing patient visits to hospital, facilitating early discharge from healthcare facility, and minimizing the unnecessary use of antibiotics contributing to increased resistance.

Neutrophil gelatinase-associated lipocalin (NGAL) is a protein belonging to the lipocalin superfamily initially found in activated neutrophils. It is an intrinsic antibacterial factor. Many types of cells, including the kidney tubule, may produce NGAL in response to various injuries. It is an emerging and promising marker in clinical nephrology. Studies have revealed that severe acute peritonitis is associated with an increase of NGAL levels both in plasma and PD effluent [82]. In a multivariate regression analysis model, only the WBC and peritoneal NGAL levels were independent predictors of peritonitis events. Since peritoneal NGAL concentration is influenced only by the local inflammation. NGAL estimations should be considered as a potential tool in view of standardized clinical platforms available for reliable measurement in plasma, urine, and other fluids [83–85].

Further follow-up and case-controlled studies are needed to examine the utility of all the above markers in day-today clinical practice and under various clinical situations including recurrent peritonitis, with use of dialysates like icodextrin, and in those patients with underlying chronic inflammatory disease.

4.24 Gene Sequencing

Molecular method is a useful emerging technique and is to be used in conjunction with the traditional culture method. It offers the advantage of identification of fastidious organisms like some fungi and in situations where there is lack of growth in culture or an unculturable organism is the causative agent. However, it requires some degree of expertise and specific equipment along with interpretative skills.

A well-established tool for rapid identification of bacterial species is 16S ribosomal RNA (rRNA) gene sequencing and is now being increasingly applied for detection directly from clinical samples and for species identification from growth of colonies in culture when the species identification is inconclusive. The 16S rRNA gene is highly conserved in different species of bacteria, yet it has a few targeted hypervariable regions that provide a species-specific sequence useful for identification. The gene is stable to mutation and this property is of immense value for its clinical application. The 16S rRNA gene sequence of almost all common bacterial pathogens has been mapped and is readily available in the gene bank. Historically, it works on the principle that sequences of > 95% identity represent the same genus and sequences of > 97% identity represent the same species [86–88].

Sheela Devi et al. evaluated the role of 16S rRNA gene and ITS (Internal transcribed spacers) region PCR and sequencing for detecting bacterial and fungal pathogens from the dialysate of patients undergoing CAPD. Among the 58-dialysate fluids evaluated, the etiological agents were identified in 8(14%) samples by conventional culture, 28(48%) by automated culture, and 47(81%) by 16sS rRNA sequencing. In 23 PD fluid samples which were culture negative by both conventional and BACT/ALERT, 16sS rRNA PCR and sequencing were able to identify the pathogen. This study suggested that 16sS rRNA detection can be effectively used as a supplementary test to the culture method and for the diagnosis in culture negative peritonitis. [89].

Third-generation technologies with high-throughput sequencing of the entire 16S gene are a powerful diagnostic tool. Circular consensus sequencing combined with sophisticated denoising algorithms to remove PCR and sequencing error now makes possible to discriminate between millions of sequence reads that differ by as little as one nucleotide across the entire gene. With these technological and methodological advances, it is possible to discriminate the 16S gene and realize the full potential as a unique fingerprinting technology for pathogen identification [90].

More recently, multiplex PCR and RT-PCR help in broad range testing based on panels of suspected pathogens. PCR–electrospray ionization mass spectrometry (PCR-ESI/MS) has emerged as a technology capable of identifying nearly all known human pathogens either from microbial isolates or directly from clinical specimens. Assay primers are strategically designed to target one or more of the broad pathogen categories: bacterial, mycobacterial, fungal, or viral [91].

Real-time PCR monitors the amplification of a targeted DNA molecule during the PCR (i.e., in real time), not at its end, as in conventional PCR. It can be used to quantify nucleic acids. Quantitative real-time polymerase chain reaction is a technique useful in estimating the microbial load in any sample. This technology is clinically useful in cases of "no growth" peritonitis and to identify those patients likely to relapse despite apparent clinical improvement with standard antibiotic therapy. With this method, it may be possible to discriminate the pathogen from a contaminant by establishing critical cut off loads in samples. [92].

For mycobacterial identification by rapid means, the real-time PCR-based GeneXpert automated system can be used. This is a cartridge-based closed system for rapid identification of mycobacterium tuberculosis in clinical samples with a turnaround time of about an hour. Besides the identification of MTB in the sample, information on rifampicin resistance and resistance to other second-line drugs can also be obtained. The sensitivity and specificity of this technique in diagnosing TB peritonitis in CAPD patients is yet unknown. Where available it can be used, since if detected early, targeted treatment and catheter removal can be undertaken [93].

MALDI-TOF MS is an alternative to the 16S rRNA gene once the growth occurs in culture. Several investigators have explored its utility in identification of pathogen once the automated culture bottle is flagged as positive. The sample preparation is more tedious for direct identification from positive flagged bottles, but the identification time is shortened by several hours. The quick identification of organism even if without antimicrobial susceptibilities could help clinicians make patient-tailored treatment more accurately. Menglan Zhou et al. opined that the modified method of testing from the culture bottles had an overall equal or even better performance for yeasts and better performance for GN bacteria than GP bacteria. [94].

4.25 Recent Developments in Predicting Relapses/Assess Response to Treatment

Bacteria-derived DNA fragments and bacterial endotoxin are implicated as possible predictors. Peritoneal effluent samples collected during the course of relapsing or recurrent peritonitis episodes have significantly higher levels of bacterial DNA fragment than those without relapsing or recurrence, both 5 days before and on the day of the completion of antibiotics. Further, when bacterial DNA fragments are tested and are detectable by 34 PCR cycles 5 days before the completion of antibiotics is used as the cut-off, the test has a sensitivity of 88.9% and specificity of 60.5% for the prediction of relapsing or recurrent peritonitis [95].

Bacterial endotoxins found in the outer membrane of gram-negative bacteria are members of a class of phospholipids called lipopolysaccharides (LPS). LPS are not exogenous products of gram-negative bacteria but get released from bacteria after death and lysis of the bacterial cell. Dialysate bacterial endotoxin can be used as a prognostic indicator for treatment failure in peritonitis. In peritonitis caused by gram-negative bacteria, a detectable peritoneal endotoxin level on day 5 has a sensitivity of 66.7% and a specificity of 83.3% for predicting primary treatment failure. Strikingly, peritoneal leukocyte counts of >1000/mm^3 on day 5 had a highly superior sensitivity of 88.9% and a specificity of 89.1%. However, there was no significant difference in the endotoxin level between completed cured patients and those who relapsed [96]. Studies have shown that a detectable peritoneal endotoxin 5 days after antibiotic therapy is a pointer to primary treatment failure in peritonitis caused by gram-negative organisms, although it was inferior to peritoneal WBC count.

Using WBC count of >1090/mm^3 on day 3 as the cut-off, the sensitivity and specificity are 75% and 74%, respectively, for the prediction of treatment failure. Overall, four predictors of treatment failure have been identified that include diabetes, systolic blood pressure of <90 mmHg at presentation, dialysate leucocyte count of 1000/mm^3 on days 3 to 4, and a count of >100/mm^3 on day 5 [97]. A risk scoring system from 0 to 11.5 has been formulated with the above predictors. Diabetes (1 score), systolic blood pressure of <90 mmHg at presentation (2.5 score), dialysate leucocyte count of 1000/mm^3 on days 3 to 4 (1.5 score), and a count of >100/mm3 on day 5 (6.5 score). This can be adopted by caregivers for determining the outcomes of treatment [5].

4.26 Future Directions and Use of Algorithms Based on Artificial Intelligence

The emerging concept of "immune fingerprinting" and the development of artificial intelligence (AI)-assisted pattern recognition of these fingerprints through machine learning algorithms is a current novel approach. Immune fingerprinting is a viable and attractive adjunct in the diagnosis of peritonitis and might further promote the development of novel point-of-care diagnostic strategies in this field. Though the current ISPD diagnostic criteria for peritonitis remain reliable and indispensable, these novel diagnostic and prognostic tests are promising and could certainly have impactful clinical applications in the future if they are used as adjunct tests [98].

A panel consisting of local immune cells, inflammatory and regulatory cytokines and chemokines, and tissue damage-related factors that would constitute specific immune fingerprints for various pathogens are used to derive algorithms. Distinct profiles of immunological and inflammatory markers discriminate gram-positive and gram-negative organisms. They can be specifically used as markers in culture-negative peritonitis also. For instance, the combination of IL-15, IL-16, and soluble IL-6 receptor levels, total cell count, and MMP substrate turnover is associated with coagulase-negative *Staphylococcus* infections, whereas a pattern of IL-1 beta, IL-15, MMP substrate, tumor necrosis factor-beta, and zymography is associated with enterococcal infection. Thus, pathogen-specific diagnosis in PD patients with highly predictive modeling is a future tool and a valuable diagnostic aid. Collection and analysis of a large volume of data with artificial intelligence-based diagnostic criteria is required for its successful application [99].

4.27 Exit Site Infection

Acute exit site infection is defined as drainage with blood and/or pus from the exit site, associated with redness (twice the size of the catheter diameter), tenderness, overgrown granulated tissue, and swelling.

Exit site infection (ESI) precedes development of tunnel infection and peritonitis. Daily exit site care can help avoid catheter infection. Exit site care and local dressing constitute the cornerstone in the management of ESI.

Typically, infection presents initially as increased crust formation and/or erythema surrounding the exit site and progresses to serous and purulent drainage arising from the site. Patients generally do not have fever or chills in the early stages of infection.

The catheter and exit site become colonized with bacteria soon after catheter placement. Bacteria secrete a biofilm, which encourages further bacterial growth and protects the colonizing organisms from antibodies, white blood cells, and antimicrobial agents.

Colonization predisposes to infection, which occurs following mild exit site trauma. The infection may involve the exit site alone or also the tunnel in which the catheter resides. A tunnel infection usually occurs only in the presence of an exit site infection.

Any drainage should be sent for Gram stain and culture to direct antibiotic therapy. The catheter tract can be milked to express drainage. Culture of the site is not helpful if drainage is not present, since, in the absence of discharge, positive cultures may just represent colonization. When cleaning the exit site, crusts, if present, should not be forcibly removed.

Routine monitoring of the exit site is essential. It should be examined daily by the patient and monthly by a clinician in order to detect infection as early as possible. In addition, the exit site should be examined by a clinician whenever the patient detects a change in the appearance of the exit site. The catheter tract should be milked to see if any drainage is present and observed for evidence of erythema overlying the tunnel.

Topical antiseptics (e.g., mupirocin, gentamicin ointment) are recommended for dressing of exit sites. Other alternatives such as hypertonic saline solution can be considered in selected cases (e.g., *P. aeruginosa*). Exit site infections have dropped significantly since the start of antimicrobial prophylaxis and other preventive measures. Povidone iodine solution (10%) and chlorhexidine solution (0.05 to 2%) have been shown to reduce the incidence of exit site infection (ESI) compared with soap and water.

Risk factors associated with development of ESI include the following [100]:

- Poor competency of exit site care
- Catheter mobilization
- Catheter pulling-out injury
- Mechanical compression of the catheter by a waist belt
- Swimming
- Presence of pets during exchanges
- Compression of the exit site by a peritoneal dialysis catheter bag

Exit site infections are caused by touch contamination organisms, especially gram-positive *S. aureus* and certain gram-negative bacteria like *P. aeruginosa*. However, a host of other organisms including those considered as normal flora have the potential to cause the infection. The percentage caused by *Staphylococcus aureus* appears to have decreased with relative increases in other gram-positive organisms and gram-negative organisms. Non-tuberculous mycobacteria, *Corynebacterium* species and yeasts are some of the emerging organisms implicated in ESI. The relative proportion of fungal infections has increased with prophylactic use of antibiotic.

Organisms causing exit site infection are as follows [101]

Total episodes 1194	
Gram-positive	79%
Coagulase-negative staphylococci	23%
Staphylococcus aureus	29%
Streptococcus species	6%
Gram-negatives	7%
Fungal	0.6&

4.28 Tunnel Infections

A tunnel infection is diagnosed when there is erythema or tenderness or swelling over the peritoneal dialysis subcutaneous tunnel pathway. Many patients who have exit site infections will also have a tunnel infection that is occult and can only be diagnosed with certainty by an ultrasound of the tunnel. An ultrasound of the catheter is undertaken if there is a suspicion of a tunnel abscess based on symptoms and physical or if ESI is resistant to treatment. It is effective in revealing fluid collections.

Tunnel involvement manifests as erythema, oedema, induration, or tenderness over the catheter pathway. If untreated, infection may progress to abscess formation within the tunnel. Tunnel abscess is more likely with infections caused by *S. aureus* or *P. aeruginosa*.

4.29 Important Points

- Peritonitis in PD may be directly related to peritoneal dialysis, due to contamination with commensal or pathogenic skin bacteria during exchanges or to an exit site or tunnel infection, or secondary to a non-dialysis-related intra-abdominal or systemic process. Most cases are peritoneal dialysis-related.
- The common symptoms are abdominal pain and cloudy peritoneal effluent. In APD, cloudy fluid may not be evident. Physical exam reveals abdominal tenderness, rebound tenderness, and occasionally systemic signs, including hypotension.
- In all suspected persons, peritoneal fluid should be sent for cell count and differential, gram stain and culture. Culture of any purulent drainage from the exit site should be performed. If accompanied by sepsis, blood cell counts and cultures should be done. Transport time of sample to the laboratory has to be minimized.
- The first cloudy bag before the start of antibiotics is the best specimen.
- In case of delay in submission of the bag to the laboratory, it is to be refrigerated at 4° to 8 ° C.

- The PD fluid is subjected to centrifugation, washing concentration method to obtain the yield in culture.
- If the peritonitis has not clinically improved at day 3 or cultures are persistently negative in spite of clinical signs and symptoms, special culture/diagnostic techniques for Mycobacteria, Nocardia, Legionella, filamentous fungus, or other fastidious bacteria should be considered.
- Empiric antibiotic regimens should be center-specific and cover both Gram-positive and Gram-negative organisms.
- In relapsing or refractory peritonitis, Mycobacteria, fungus, and exit or tunnel infections should be ruled out.
- For tuberculous peritonitis, molecular assays offer a distinct advantage in terms of better sensitivity, rapid turnaround time, and information on anti-tuberculous drug susceptibility. They should be considered in all cases of suspected tuberculous peritonitis over and above the conventional techniques.
- Newer diagnostic methods of diagnosis including molecular testing and automated techniques have good sensitivity with better turnaround times. They should be sought where feasible for diagnostic work up in culture negative peritonitis especially in tuberculous peritonitis or peritonitis caused by fastidious/non-cultivable bacteria.

References

1. El-Reshaid W, Al-Disawy H, Nassef H, Alhelaly U. Comparison of peritonitis rates and patient survival in automated and continuous ambulatory peritoneal dialysis: a 10-year single center experience. Ren Fail. 2016;38(8):1187–92. https://doi.org/10.1080/0886022X.2016.1209025.
2. Kaene WF, Vas SI. Peritonitis Chapter 16. In: Gokal R, Nolph KD, editors. The textbook of peritoneal dialysis. 1st ed. Kluwer: Academic Publishers; 1994.
3. Tzamaloukas AH, Obermiller LE, Gibel LJ, et al. Peritonitis associated with intra-abdominal pathology in continuous ambulatory peritoneal dialysis patients. Perit Dial Int. 1993;13(Suppl 2):S335–7.
4. Li PK, Szeto CC, Piraino B, et al. ISPD peritonitis recommendations: 2016 update on prevention and treatment [published correction appears in Perit Dial Int. 2018 Jul-Aug;38(4):313]. Perit Dial Int. 2016;36(5):481–508. https://doi.org/10.3747/pdi.2016.00078.
5. Nochaiwong S, Ruengorn C, Koyratkoson K, et al. A clinical risk prediction tool for peritonitis-associated treatment failure in peritoneal dialysis patients. Sci Rep. 2018;8(1):14797. https://doi.org/10.1038/s41598-018-33196-2.
6. Ghali JR, Bannister KM, Brown FG, et al. Microbiology and outcomes of peritonitis in Australian peritoneal dialysis patients. Perit Dial Int. 2011;31(6):651–62. https://doi.org/10.3747/pdi.2010.00131.
7. Manera KE, Johnson DW, Craig JC, et al. Patient and caregiver priorities for outcomes in peritoneal dialysis: multinational nominal group technique study. Clin J Am Soc Nephrol. 2019;14(1):74–83. https://doi.org/10.2215/CJN.05380518.
8. Salzer WL. Peritoneal dialysis-related peritonitis: challenges and solutions. Int J Nephrol Renovasc Dis. 2018;11:173–86. https://doi.org/10.2147/IJNRD.S123618.
9. Wang HH, Huang CH, Kuo MC, et al. Microbiology of peritoneal dialysis-related infection and factors of refractory peritoneal dialysis related peritonitis: a ten-year single-center

study in Taiwan. J Microbiol Immunol Infect. 2019;52(5):752–9. https://doi.org/10.1016/j.jmii.2018.10.013.
10. Prasad N, Gupta A, Sharma RK, Prasad KN, Gulati S, Sharma AP. Outcome of gram-positive and gram-negative peritonitis in patients on continuous ambulatory peritoneal dialysis: a single-center experience. Perit Dial Int. 2003;23(Suppl 2):S144–7.
11. Pindi G, Kawle V, Sunkara RR, Darbha MS, Garikaparthi S. Continuous ambulatory peritoneal dialysis peritonitis: microbiology and outcomes. Indian J Med Microbiol. 2020;38(1):72–7. https://doi.org/10.4103/ijmm.IJMM_20_251.
12. Kim DK, Yoo TH, Ryu DR, et al. Changes in causative organisms and their antimicrobial susceptibilities in CAPD peritonitis: a single center's experience over one decade. Perit Dial Int. 2004;24(5):424–32.
13. Mujais S. Microbiology and outcomes of peritonitis in North America. Kidney Int Suppl. 2006;103:S55–62. https://doi.org/10.1038/sj.ki.5001916.
14. Kan GW, Thomas MA, Heath CH. A 12-month review of peritoneal dialysis-related peritonitis in Western Australia: is empiric vancomycin still indicated for some patients? Perit Dial Int. 2003;23(5):465–8.
15. Port FK, Held PJ, Nolph KD, Turenne MN, Wolfe RA. Risk of peritonitis and technique failure by CAPD connection technique: a national study. Kidney Int. 1992;42(4):967–74. https://doi.org/10.1038/ki.1992.375.
16. Bunke M, Brier ME, Golper TA. Culture-negative CAPD peritonitis: the network 9 study. Adv Perit Dial. 1994;10:174–8.
17. Mushahar L, Mei LW, Yusuf WS, Sivathasan S, Kamaruddin N, Idzham NJ. Exit-site dressing and infection in peritoneal dialysis: a randomized controlled pilot trial. Perit Dial Int. 2016;36(2):135–9. https://doi.org/10.3747/pdi.2014.00195.
18. Szeto CC. The new ISPD peritonitis guideline. Ren Replace Ther. 2018;4:7. https://doi.org/10.1186/s41100-018-0150-2.
19. Wu G, Khanna R, Vas SI, Oreopoulos DG. Is extensive diverticulosis of the colon a contraindication for CAPD? Perit Dial Bull. 1983;3(4):180–3.
20. Machuca E, Ortiz AM, Rabagliati R. Streptococcus viridans-associated peritonitis after gastroscopy. Adv Perit Dial. 2005;21:60–2.
21. Bakan A, Oral A, Kostek O, Ecder SA, Odabaş AR. An unusual case of peritonitis after vaginal leak in a patient on peritoneal dialysis. Nefrologia. 2016;36(1):85–6. https://doi.org/10.1016/j.nefro.2015.08.006.
22. Hakim A, Hisam N, Reuman PD. Environmental mycobacterial peritonitis complicating peritoneal dialysis: three cases and review. Clin Infect Dis. 1993;16(3):426–31. https://doi.org/10.1093/clind/16.3.426.
23. Dasgupta MK, Anwar H, Costerton JW. Bacterial biofilms and peritonitis in continuos ambulatory peritoneal dialysis. Int Biodeterior Biodegradation. 1992;30:167–76.
24. Martins M, Rodrigues A, Pedrosa JM, Carvalho MJ, Cabrita A, Oliveira R. Update on the challenging role of biofilms in peritoneal dialysis. Biofouling. 2013;29(8):1015–27. https://doi.org/10.1080/08927014.2013.824566.
25. Tan R, Weng W, Raymond WD, Sieunarine K. Outcomes in buried versus non-buried peritoneal dialysis catheters: a retrospective cohort study. J Vasc Access. 2021;22(2):254–60. https://doi.org/10.1177/1129729820937111.
26. Demoulin N, Goffin E. Intraperitoneal urokinase and oral rifampicin for persisting asymptomatic dialysate infection following acute coagulase-negative staphylococcus peritonitis. Perit Dial Int. 2009;29(5):548–53.
27. Wong SS, Lau WY, Chan PK, Wan CK, Cheng YL. Extended experience in the use of antibiotic lock for eradication of biofilm bacteria on Tenckhoff catheter. Perit Dial Int. 2019;39(2):187–90. https://doi.org/10.3747/pdi.2018.00098.
28. Tian Y, Xie X, Xiang S, et al. Risk factors and outcomes of early-onset peritonitis in Chinese peritoneal dialysis patients. Kidney Blood Press Res. 2017;42(6):1266–76. https://doi.org/10.1159/000485930.

29. Fieren MW. The local inflammatory responses to infection of the peritoneal cavity in humans: their regulation by cytokines, macrophages, and other leukocytes. Mediat Inflamm. 2012;2012:976241. https://doi.org/10.1155/2012/976241.
30. Flanigan MJ, Freeman RM, Lim VS. Cellular response to peritonitis among peritoneal dialysis patients. Am J Kidney Dis. 1985;6(6):420–4. https://doi.org/10.1016/s0272-6386(85)80105-0.
31. Charney DI, Gouge SF. Chemical peritonitis secondary to intraperitoneal vancomycin. Am J Kidney Dis. 1991;17(1):76–9. https://doi.org/10.1016/s0272-6386(12)80255-1.
32. Streather CP, Carr P, Barton IK. Carcinoma of the kidney presenting as sterile peritonitis in a patient on continuous ambulatory peritoneal dialysis. Nephron. 1991;58(1):121. https://doi.org/10.1159/000186395.
33. Bargman JM, Zent R, Ellis P, Auger M, Wilson S. Diagnosis of lymphoma in a continuous ambulatory peritoneal dialysis patient by peritoneal fluid cytology. Am J Kidney Dis. 1994;23(5):747–50. https://doi.org/10.1016/s0272-6386(12)70289-5.
34. Tintillier M, Pochet JM, Christophe JL, Scheiff JM, Goffin E. Transient sterile chemical peritonitis with icodextrin: clinical presentation, prevalence, and literature review. Perit Dial Int. 2002;22(4):534–7.
35. Ejaz AA, Fitzpatrick PM, Durkin AJ, et al. Pathophysiology of peritoneal fluid eosinophilia in peritoneal dialysis patients. Nephron. 1999;81(2):125–30. https://doi.org/10.1159/000045266.
36. Lew SQ. Hemoperitoneum: bloody peritoneal dialysate in ESRD patients receiving peritoneal dialysis. Perit Dial Int. 2007;27(3):226–33.
37. Prasad KN. Peritonitis in patients on continuous ambulatory peritoneal dialysis: a brief microbiological review. Ind J Peritoneal Dialysis. 1999;2:12–7.
38. Amici G, Grandesso S, Mottola A, Virga G, Calconi G, Bocci C. Fungal peritonitis in peritoneal dialysis: critical review of six cases. Adv Perit Dial. 1994;10:169–73.
39. Stuck A, Seiler A, Frey FJ. Peritonitis due to an intrauterine contraceptive device in a patient on CAPD. Perit Dial Bull. 1986;6:158–9.
40. Ozeki T, Mizuno M, Iguchi D, et al. C1 inhibitor mitigates peritoneal injury in zymosan-induced peritonitis. Am J Physiol Renal Physiol. 2021;320(6):F1123–32. https://doi.org/10.1152/ajprenal.00600.2020.
41. Santos ACMLD, ACM M, Barbosa TA, et al. Phenotypic and molecular characterization of nonfermenting gram-negative bacilli causing peritonitis in peritoneal dialysis patients. Pathogens. 2022;11(2):218. https://doi.org/10.3390/pathogens11020218.
42. Talwani R, Horvath JA. Tuberculous peritonitis in patients undergoing continuous ambulatory peritoneal dialysis: case report and review. Clin Infect Dis. 2000;31(1):70–5. https://doi.org/10.1086/313919.
43. Lin JH, Wang WJ, Yang HY, et al. Non-tuberculous and tuberculous mycobacterial peritonitis in peritoneal dialysis patients. Ren Fail. 2014;36(7):1158–61. https://doi.org/10.3109/0886022X.2014.918842.
44. Abraham G, Mathews M, Sekar L, Srikanth A, Sekar U, Soundarajan P. Tuberculous peritonitis in a cohort of continuous ambulatory peritoneal dialysis patients. Perit Dial Int. 2001;21(Suppl 3):S202–4.
45. Muthucumarana K, Howson P, Crawford D, Burrows S, Swaminathan R, Irish A. The relationship between presentation and the time of initial Administration of Antibiotics with Outcomes of peritonitis in peritoneal dialysis patients: the PROMPT study. Kidney Int Rep. 2016;1(2):65–72. https://doi.org/10.1016/j.ekir.2016.05.003.
46. Oliveira LG, Luengo J, Caramori JC, Montelli AC, Cunha Mde L, Barretti P. Peritonitis in recent years: clinical findings and predictors of treatment response of 170 episodes at a single Brazilian center. Int Urol Nephrol. 2012;44(5):1529–37. https://doi.org/10.1007/s11255-011-0107-7.
47. Voinescu CG, Khanna R. Peritonitis in peritoneal dialysis. Int J Artif Organs. 2002;25(4):249–60. https://doi.org/10.1177/039139880202500402.

48. Barretti P, Montelli AC, Batalha JE, Caramori JC, Cunha ML. The role of virulence factors in the outcome of staphylococcal peritonitis in CAPD patients. BMC Infect Dis. 2009;9:212. https://doi.org/10.1186/1471-2334-9-212.
49. Clements TW, Tolonen M, Ball CG, Kirkpatrick AW. Secondary peritonitis and intra-abdominal sepsis: an increasingly global disease in search of better systemic therapies. Scand J Surg. 2021;110(2):139–49. https://doi.org/10.1177/1457496920984078.
50. Al Sahlawi M, Bargman JM, Perl J. Peritoneal dialysis-associated peritonitis: suggestions for management and mistakes to avoid. Kidney Med. 2020;2(4):467–75. https://doi.org/10.1016/j.xkme.2020.04.010.
51. Taylor PM. Image-guided peritoneal access and management of complications in peritoneal dialysis. Semin Dial. 2002;15(4):250–8. https://doi.org/10.1046/j.1525-139x.2002.00067.x.
52. Trinh E, Saiprasertkit N, Bargman JM. Increased serum lactate in peritoneal dialysis patients presenting with Intercurrent illness. Perit Dial Int. 2018;38(5):363–5. https://doi.org/10.3747/pdi.2017.00169.
53. Yap DY, Chu WL, Ng F, Yip TP, Lui SL, Lo WK. Risk factors and outcome of contamination in patients on peritoneal dialysis–a single-center experience of 15 years. Perit Dial Int. 2012 Nov-Dec;32(6):612–6. https://doi.org/10.3747/pdi.2011.00268.
54. Johnson DW, Gray N, Snelling P. A peritoneal dialysis patient with fatal culture-negative peritonitis. Nephrology (Carlton). 2003;8(1):49–55. https://doi.org/10.1046/j.1440-1797.2003.00119.x.
55. von Graevenitz A, Amsterdam D. Microbiological aspects of peritonitis associated with continuous ambulatory peritoneal dialysis. Clin Microbiol Rev. 1992;5(1):36–48. https://doi.org/10.1128/CMR.5.1.36.
56. Park M-S, Yoo IY, Kang O-K, Lee JE, Kim DJ, Huh HJ, Lee NY. Evaluation of BacT/Alert FAN plus bottles for the culture of peritoneal dialysate. Annals of clinical. Microbiology. 2019;22(4):90–5.
57. Htay H, Cho Y, Pascoe EM, et al. Multicentre registry data analysis comparing outcomes of culture-negative peritonitis and different subtypes of culture-positive peritonitis in peritoneal dialysis patients. Perit Dial Int. 2020;40(1):47–56. https://doi.org/10.1177/0896860819879891.
58. Karanicolas S, Oreopoulos DG, Izatt S, et al. Epidemic of aseptic peritonitis caused by endotoxin during chronic peritoneal dialysis. N Engl J Med. 1977;296(23):1336–7. https://doi.org/10.1056/NEJM197706092962309.
59. Teitelbaum I. Cloudy peritoneal dialysate: it's not always infection. Contrib Nephrol. 2006;150:187–94. https://doi.org/10.1159/000093594.
60. Oh SY, Kim H, Kang JM, et al. Eosinophilic peritonitis in a patient with continuous ambulatory peritoneal dialysis (CAPD). Korean J Intern Med. 2004;19(2):121–3. https://doi.org/10.3904/kjim.2004.19.2.121.
61. Enríquez J, Klínger J, Arturo JA, Tobar C, Ceballos O. Immunophenotyping by flow cytometry of peritoneal fluid of patients with peritonitis on continuous ambulatory peritoneal dialysis. Adv Perit Dial. 2002;18:184–7.
62. Dong J, Li Z, Xu R, Chen Y, Luo S, Li Y. Disease severity score could not predict the outcomes in peritoneal dialysis-associated peritonitis. Nephrol Dial Transplant. 2012;27(6):2496–501. https://doi.org/10.1093/ndt/gfr654.
63. Chu G. A defined peritonitis clinical pathway in the emergency department improves outcomes for peritoneal dialysis patients. Renal Society of Australasia Journal. 2014;10(1):30–3.
64. Prasad KN, Singh K, Rizwan A, et al. Microbiology and outcomes of peritonitis in northern India. Perit Dial Int. 2014;34(2):188–94. https://doi.org/10.3747/pdi.2012.00233.
65. Nessim SJ, Nisenbaum R, Bargman JM, Jassal SV. Microbiology of peritonitis in peritoneal dialysis patients with multiple episodes. Perit Dial Int. 2012;32(3):316–21. https://doi.org/10.3747/pdi.2011.00058.
66. Bieber SD, Anderson AE, Mehrotra R. Diagnostic testing for peritonitis in patients undergoing peritoneal dialysis. Semin Dial. 2014;27:602–6. https://doi.org/10.1111/sdi.12270.

67. Sekar U, Suppiah R, Abraham G, Mathew M, Padma G, Shroff S, Soundarajan P. Does the method of sampling influence microbiological diagnosis of peritonitis in CAPD? Indian J Perit Dial. 1999;2:18–24.
68. Forbes BA, Frymoyer PA, Kopecky RT, Wojtaszek JM, Pettit DJ. Evaluation of the lysis-centrifugation system for culturing dialysates from continuous ambulatory peritoneal dialysis patients with peritonitis. Am J Kidney Dis. 1988;11(2):176–9. https://doi.org/10.1016/s0272-6386(88)80208-7.
69. Kanjanabuch T, Chatsuwan T, Udomsantisuk N, et al. Association of Local Unit Sampling and Microbiology Laboratory Culture Practices with the ability to identify causative pathogens in peritoneal dialysis-associated peritonitis in Thailand. Kidney Int Rep. 2021;6(4):1118–29. https://doi.org/10.1016/j.ekir.2021.01.010.
70. Lin WH, Hwang JC, Tseng CC, et al. Matrix-assisted laser desorption ionization-time of flight mass spectrometry accelerates pathogen identification and may confer benefit in the outcome of peritoneal dialysis-related peritonitis. J Clin Microbiol. 2016;54(5):1381–3. https://doi.org/10.1128/JCM.03378-153.
71. Chegou NN, Hoek KG, Kriel M, Warren RM, Victor TC, Walzl G. Tuberculosis assays: past, present and future. Expert Rev Anti-Infect Ther. 2011;9(4):457–69. https://doi.org/10.1586/eri.11.23.
72. Bezerra DA, Silva MB, Caramori JS, et al. The diagnostic value of gram stain for initial identification of the etiologic agent of peritonitis in CAPD patients. Perit Dial Int. 1997;17(3):269–72.
73. Lye WC. Rapid diagnosis of mycobacterium tuberculous peritonitis in two continuous ambulatory peritoneal dialysis patients, using DNA amplification by polymerase chain reaction. Adv Perit Dial. 2002;18:154–7.
74. Li PK, Szeto CC, Piraino B, et al. Peritoneal dialysis-related infections recommendations: 2010 update [published correction appears in Perit Dial Int. 2011 Sep-Oct;31(5):512]. Perit Dial Int. 2010;30(4):393–423. https://doi.org/10.3747/pdi.2010.00049.
75. Vaz S. Laboratory diagnosis of peritonitis in peritoneal dialysis patients? Indian J Perit Dial. 1999;2:8–11.
76. Twardowski ZJ, Prowant BF. Classification of normal and diseased exit sites. Perit Dial Int. 1996;16(Suppl 3):S32–50.
77. Sangeetha B, Deepa N, Hemalatha M, Latha CM, Ram R, Kumar VS. Exit-site infection: a comparison of classification systems. Perit Dial Int. 2018;38(6):462–3. https://doi.org/10.3747/pdi.2018.00013.
78. Fung WW, Li PK. Recent advances in novel diagnostic testing for peritoneal dialysis-related peritonitis. Kidney Res Clin Pract. 2022;41(2):156–64. https://doi.org/10.23876/j.krcp.21.204.
79. Rathore V, Joshi H, Kimmatkar PD, et al. Leukocyte esterase reagent strip as a bedside tool to detect peritonitis in patients undergoing acute peritoneal dialysis. Saudi J Kidney Dis Transpl. 2017;28(6):1264–9. https://doi.org/10.4103/1319-2442.220875.
80. Goodlad C, George S, Sandoval S, et al. Measurement of innate immune response biomarkers in peritoneal dialysis effluent using a rapid diagnostic point-of-care device as a diagnostic indicator of peritonitis. Kidney Int. 2020;97(6):1253–9. https://doi.org/10.1016/j.kint.2020.01.044.
81. Atkinson SJ, Nolan M, Klingbeil L, et al. Intestine-derived matrix Metalloproteinase-8 is a critical mediator of Polymicrobial peritonitis. Crit Care Med. 2016;44(4):e200–6. https://doi.org/10.1097/CCM.0000000000001374.
82. Devarajan P. Neutrophil gelatinase-associated lipocalin (NGAL): a new marker of kidney disease. Scand J Clin Lab Invest Suppl. 2008;241:89–94. https://doi.org/10.1080/00365510802150158.
83. Leung JC, Lam MF, Tang SC, et al. Roles of neutrophil gelatinase-associated lipocalin in continuous ambulatory peritoneal dialysis-related peritonitis. J Clin Immunol. 2009;29(3):365–78. https://doi.org/10.1007/s10875-008-9271-7.

84. Lacquaniti A, Chirico V, Mondello S, et al. Neutrophil gelatinase-associated lipocalin in peritoneal dialysis reflects status of peritoneum. J Nephrol. 2013;26(6):1151–9. https://doi.org/10.5301/jn.5000271.
85. Devarajan P. Neutrophil gelatinase-associated lipocalin (NGAL): a new marker of kidney disease. Scand J Clin Lab Invest. 2008;68(sup241):89–94. https://doi.org/10.1080/00365510802150158.
86. Patel JB. 16S rRNA gene sequencing for bacterial pathogen identification in the clinical laboratory. Mol Diagn. 2001;6(4):313–21. https://doi.org/10.1054/modi.2001.29158.
87. Petti CA. Detection and identification of microorganisms by gene amplification and sequencing. Clin Infect Dis. 2007;44(8):1108–14. https://doi.org/10.1086/512818.
88. Johnson JS, Spakowicz DJ, Hong BY, Petersen LM, Demkowicz P, Chen L, Leopold SR, Hanson BM, Agresta HO, Gerstein M, Sodergren E, Weinstock GM. Evaluation of 16S rRNA gene sequencing for species and strain-level microbiome analysis. Nat Commun. 2019 Nov 6;10(1):5029. https://doi.org/10.1038/s41467-019-13036-1.
89. Sheela Devi C, Vivian Joseph Ratnam P, Ramya SR, et al. Detection of 16S rRNA gene for rapid identification of bacterial pathogens causing peritonitis in patients on continuous ambulatory peritoneal dialysis [published online ahead of print, 2022 Apr 20]. Indian J Med Microbiol. 2022;S0255-0857(22):00056–1. https://doi.org/10.1016/j.ijmmb.2022.03.011.
90. Lao HY, Ng TT, Wong RY, Wong CS, Lee LK, Wong DS, Chan CT, Jim SH, Leung JS, Lo HW, Wong IT, Yau MC, Lam JY, Wu AK, Siu GK. The clinical utility of two high-throughput 16S rRNA gene sequencing workflows for taxonomic assignment of unidentifiable bacterial pathogens in matrix-assisted laser desorption ionization-time of flight mass spectrometry. J Clin Microbiol. 2022 Jan 19;60(1):e0176921. https://doi.org/10.1128/JCM.01769-21.
91. Wolk DM, Kaleta EJ, Wysocki VH. PCR-electrospray ionization mass spectrometry: the potential to change infectious disease diagnostics in clinical and public health laboratories. J Mol Diagn. 2012;14(4):295–304. https://doi.org/10.1016/j.jmoldx.2012.02.005.
92. Johnson G, Wilks M, Warwick S, Millar MR, Fan SL. Comparative study of diagnosis of PD peritonitis by quantitative polymerase chain reaction for bacterial DNA vs culture methods. J Nephrol. 2006;19(1):45–9.
93. Edwards S, Glynn P, David MD, Kamesh L. Diagnosing tuberculous peritonitis early in patients on peritoneal dialysis: use of Xpert MTB/RIF assay. Perit Dial Int. 2016;36(4):461–3. https://doi.org/10.3747/pdi.2015.00233.
94. Zhou M, Yang Q, Kudinha T, et al. An improved in-house MALDI-TOF MS protocol for direct cost-effective identification of pathogens from blood cultures. Front Microbiol. 2017;8:1824. https://doi.org/10.3389/fmicb.2017.01824.
95. Szeto CC, Lai KB, Kwan BC, et al. Bacteria-derived DNA fragment in peritoneal dialysis effluent as a predictor of relapsing peritonitis. Clin J Am Soc Nephrol. 2013;8(11):1935–41. https://doi.org/10.2215/CJN.02360213.
96. Szeto CC, Lai KB, Chow KM, et al. Dialysate bacterial endotoxin as a prognostic indicator of peritoneal dialysis related peritonitis. Nephrology (Carlton). 2016;21(12):1069–72. https://doi.org/10.1111/nep.12828.
97. Chow KM, Szeto CC, Cheung KK, et al. Predictive value of dialysate cell counts in peritonitis complicating peritoneal dialysis. Clin J Am Soc Nephrol. 2006;1(4):768–73. https://doi.org/10.2215/CJN.01010306.
98. Takeuchi T, Ohno H, Satoh-Takayama N. Understanding the immune signature fingerprint of peritoneal dialysis-related peritonitis. Kidney Int. 2017;92(1):16–8. https://doi.org/10.1016/j.kint.2017.02.027.
99. Zhang J, Friberg IM, Kift-Morgan A, et al. Machine-learning algorithms define pathogen-specific local immune fingerprints in peritoneal dialysis patients with bacterial infections. Kidney Int. 2017;92(1):179–91. https://doi.org/10.1016/j.kint.2017.01.017.

100. Lin J, Ye H, Li J, et al. Prevalence and risk factors of exit-site infection in incident peritoneal dialysis patients. Perit Dial Int. 2020;40(2):164–70. https://doi.org/10.1177/0896860819886965.
101. Nessim SJ, Komenda P, Rigatto C, Verrelli M, Sood MM. Frequency and microbiology of peritonitis and exit-site infection among obese peritoneal dialysis patients. Perit Dial Int. 2013;33(2):167–74. https://doi.org/10.3747/pdi.2011.00244.
102. https://www.azuravascularcare.com/infodialysisaccess/peritonitis-related-to-peritoneal-dialysis, Aug 23, 2019.

Medical Management of Peritonitis with Antimicrobial Therapy

5

Santosh Varughese, Phanidhar Mogga, and Priya Anantharaman

A 40-year-old gentleman with end-stage kidney disease due to IgA nephropathy has been on continuous ambulatory peritoneal dialysis for 2 years. He presented with abdominal pain, feverishness, and watery loose stools for 2 days. This morning, his PD fluid effluent is turbid. A preemptive diagnosis of PD peritonitis was made. The PD fluid counts were 13,000/ml and the gram stain was negative. He was started on empiric antibiotic therapy.

5.1 Diagnosis and Identification of the Infective Organism

All patients presenting with cloudy PD fluid effluent are presumed to have peritonitis, though other conditions may mimic the presentation of peritonitis; e.g., chemical peritonitis, PD fluid sample collected from a "dry" abdomen, hemoperitoneum, presence of malignant cells, or due to fibrin or triglycerides in the PD fluid, the latter appears milky and occurs due to calcium channel blockers, lymphatic obstruction and acute pancreatitis [1]. PD peritonitis is also one of the important differential diagnoses to be considered in the presence of abdominal pain even if the PD fluid effluent is clear. History of accidental contamination or disconnection, gastrointestinal endoscopic or gynecological procedures, or constipation or diarrhea is elicited

S. Varughese (✉)
Christian Medical College, Vellore, Tamil Nadu, India

P. Mogga
MGM Healthcare Chennai, Chennai, Tamil Nadu, India

P. Anantharaman
Jersey Coast Nephrology and Hypertension Associates, Brick Township, NJ, USA

G. Abraham et al. (eds.), *Diagnosis and Management of Complications of Peritoneal Dialysis related Peritonitis*,
https://doi.org/10.1007/978-981-99-2275-8_5

as is past history of exit site infection of peritonitis. Examination typically reveals generalized tenderness. Tenderness that is localized or presence of rebound suggests possible underlying surgical cause of peritonitis. Redness or discharge from the exit site or tenderness of fluid in the tunnel suggests infection of the respective areas.

In every patient suspected to have PD peritonitis, PD fluid effluent is drained and sent for leucocyte count—total and differential, smear and gram stain, and culture, the last to be done at least within 6 h of draining the fluid. The preferred method of culture is inoculating 5 to 10 ml either directly or by centrifugation of 50 ml of the effluent for 15 min at 3000 g and culturing the pellet after suspending 3 to 5 ml of supernatant in a BACTEC kit (rapid blood culture bottle) to increase the likelihood of growth [2, 3]. Gram stain of the PD fluid effluent is frequently negative [4, 5] but may help in early detection of fungal peritonitis thus allowing prompt initiation of therapy [6]. The fluid is also sent for fungal and mycobacterial cultures in appropriate media. The tests and cultures are repeated if the cultures are negative after 3 to 5 days of antibiotic therapy. If the catheter is removed, the intraperitoneal segment is sent for culture and the identification of enterococcal and fungal infections [7]. Peripheral blood cultures are sent in patients who are on immunosuppressive drugs [8] or are septic [9]. The presence of bacteremia in a patient with PD peritonitis suggests intrabdominal pathology [10, 11].

A diagnosis of PD peritonitis requires at least two of the following: (i) Abdominal pain and/or cloudy PD fluid effluent, i.e., clinical features suggesting peritonitis; (ii) elevated leukocyte count in the PD fluid effluent (>100/mL or > 0.1 × 10 [9]/L (following a minimum dwell of 2 h), with neutrophils constituting >50% of the leukocytes; and (iii) culture positivity of PD effluent. In patients on automated peritoneal dialysis, the presence of more than 50% of neutrophils strongly suggests PD peritonitis even if the absolute value of leucocyte count is less than 100/ml [12].

5.2 Antimicrobial Therapy

After initial PD fluid effluent samples have been obtained, empiric antimicrobial therapy is started immediately, preferably by intraperitoneal (IP) route. Intravenous (IV) antibiotics may be preferred in patients with septicemia. The risk of mortality of modality failure increases by 5.5% for each hour's delay in starting antimicrobial therapy [13], and a delay of 24 h from onset of clinical features of PD peritonitis confers a threefold likelihood of PD catheter removal [14]. The algorithm on initial evaluation and management is depicted in Fig. 5.1. Most patients with PD peritonitis can be managed as outpatients and severity of abdominal pain and systemic features guiding decision on hospital admission. Patients should follow-up within 48 to 72 h to report resolution (or lack of it) of symptoms and fluid color and for repeat fluid counts and follow-up culture reports to confirm appropriateness of choice of antibiotics.

The goal of care is "medical cure" which is said to be effective when there is complete resolution of PD peritonitis without relapse or recurrence of peritonitis, requirement of catheter removal, shift to hemodialysis for 30 days, or mortality [15].

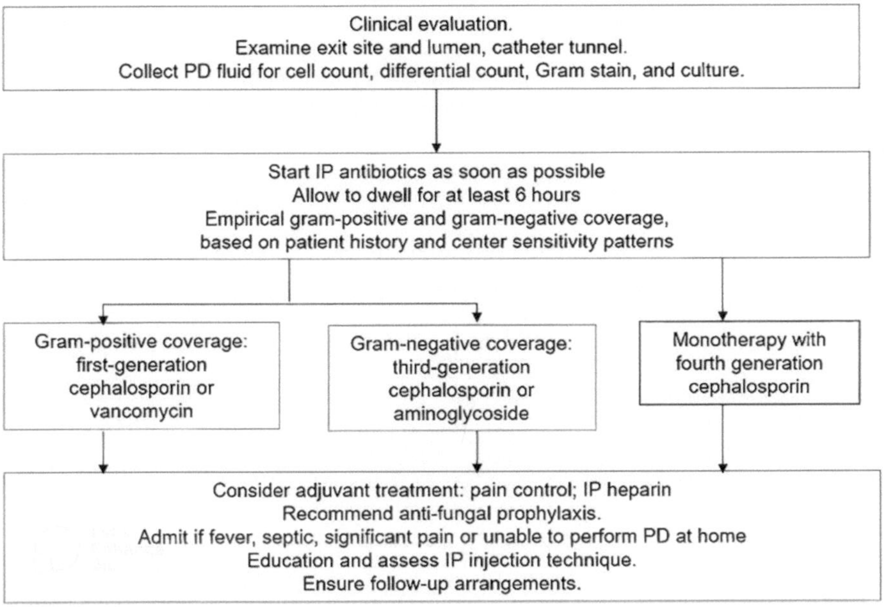

Fig. 5.1 Algorithm of evaluation and initial management of PD peritonitis [15]

The choice of initial antibiotics is based on center-specific antimicrobial susceptibility and should treat both gram-positive and gram-negative organisms. A typical choice will be a first-generation cephalosporin or vancomycin to cover gram-positive organisms and a third-generation cephalosporin or an aminoglycoside to cover gram-negative organisms. Monotherapy with cefepime may be employed to cover both gram-positive and gram-negative organisms. Prompt initiation of antimicrobial therapy results in decrease in peritoneal inflammation, pain relief, and membrane preservation.

IP cefazolin may be preferred to vancomycin to decrease likelihood of increased vancomycin resistance, while vancomycin is selected where methicillin-resistance is common [16]. Short courses of aminoglycosides may not significantly affect residual renal function [17], but oto- and vestibular toxicity remain a concern [18]. Higher cumulative doses of amikacin and vancomycin, older age group, and number of episodes of peritonitis increase the risk for hearing loss [18]. Since aminoglycosides have their maximal bactericidal activity at high peak drug concentrations, they are given once daily. These drugs continue to suppress bacterial growth at levels lower than the MIC of the bacteria (post-antibiotic effect) [19]. When cefepime monotherapy is employed, in patients with urine output more than 100 ml/day, the antibiotic dose needs to be increased by 25% to avoid underdosing [20]. Table 5.1 lists the dosing of IP antimicrobials—either *intermittent*, i.e., antibiotics are instilled in one exchange with at least 6 h dwell once daily, or *continuous*, i.e., antibiotics are instilled in each exchange. Table 5.2 lists the dosing of systemic antimicrobials – IV or oral. If fluoroquinolones are used for treatment of PD

Table 5.1 Intraperitoneal (IP) antibiotic dosing recommendations for treatment of PD peritonitis [15]

Antibiotic
Intermittent (1 exchange daily for at least 6 h)
Continuous (all exchanges)
Aminoglycosides
Amikacin
Gentamicin
Netilmicin
Tobramycin
2 mg/kg daily
0.6 mg/kg daily
0.6 mg/kg daily
0.6 mg/kg daily
Not advised
Not advised
Not advised
Not advised
Cephalosporins
Cefazolin
Cefepime
Cefoperazone
Cefotaxime
Ceftazidime
Ceftriaxone
15 mg/kg daily (long dwell)
20 mg/kg daily (short dwell)
1000 mg daily
No data
500–1000 mg daily
1000–1500 mg daily (long dwell)
20 mg/kg daily (short dwell)
1000 mg daily
LD 500 mg/L, MD 125 mg/L
LD 500 mg/L, MD 125 mg/L
LD 500 mg/L, MD 62.5–125 mg/L
No data
LD 500 mg/L, MD 125 mg/L
No data
Penicillins
Penicillin G
Amoxicillin
Ampicillin
Ampicillin/
Sulbactam
Piperacillin/
Tazobactam
Ticarcillin/
Clavulanic acid

Table 5.1 (continued)

No data
No data
4 gm daily
No data
No data
No data
LD 50,000 U/L, MD 25,000 U/L
MD 150 mg/L
MD 125 mg/L
LD 1000 mg/500 mg,
MD 133.3 mg/66.7 mg
LD 4 gm/0.5 gm,
MD 1 gm/0.125 gm
LD 3 gm/0.2 gm, MD 300 mg/20 mg/L
Others
Aztreonam
Ciprofloxacin
Clindamycin
Daptomycin
Fosfomycin
Imipenem/cilastatin
Ofloxacin
Polymyxin B
Quinupristin/
Dalfopristin
Meropenem
Teicoplanin
Vancomycin
2 gm daily
No data
No data
300 mg daily
4 g daily
500 mg in alternate exchange
No data
No data
25 mg/L in alternate exchanges
500 mg daily (long dwell APD)
1000 mg daily (short dwell CAPD)
15 mg/kg every 5 days
15–30 mg/kg every 5–7 days for CAPD
15 mg/kg every 4 days for APD
LD 500 mg/L, MD 250 mg/L
MD 50 mg/L
MD 600 mg/bag
LD 100 mg/L, MD 20 mg/L

(continued)

Table 5.1 (continued)

No data
LD 250 mg/L, MD 50 mg/L
LD 200 mg, MD 25 mg/L
MD 300,000 unit (30 mg)/bag
No data
MD 125 mg/L
LD 400 mg/bag, MD 20 mg/L
LD 20–25 mg/kg, MD 25 mg/L
Antifungal
Fluconazole
Voriconazole
IP 150–200 mg every 24 to 48 h
(Oral route is preferred; Table 5.2)
IP 2.5 mg/kg daily
(Oral route preferred; Table 5.2)
No data
No data

Table 5.2 Systemic antibiotic dosing recommendations for treatment of PD peritonitis [15]

Drug	Dosing
Antibacterial	Oral 500 mg thrice daily
Amoxicillin	Oral 500–750 mg daily
Ciprofloxacin	Oral 750 mg BD for CCPD
Clarithromycin	Oral 250 mg BD
Colistin	IV 300 mg loading (for critically ill patients), then 60–200 mg
Dalbavancin	daily
Daptomycin	IV 1500 mg over 30 min single dose
Ertapenem	IV 4–6 mg/kg every 48 h
Levofloxacin	IV 500 mg daily
Linezolid	Oral 250 mg daily or 500 mg every 48 h
Moxifloxacin	IV or oral 600 mg BD for 48 h, then 300 mg BD
Rifampicin	Oral 400 mg daily
Ticarcillin/clavulanic acid	Oral or IV 450 mg daily for BW <50 kg;
Tigecycline	600 mg daily for BW ≥50 kg
Trimethoprim/	IV 3 gm/0.2 gm every 12 h
sulfamethoxazole	IV 100 mg loading, then 50 mg every 12 h
	Oral 160 mg/800 mg BD
Anti-fungal	IV 0.75–1.0 mg/kg/day over 4–6 h
Amphotericin B	IV 3–5 mg/kg/day
deoxycholate	IV 200 mg loading, then 100 mg daily
Amphotericin B (liposomal)	IV 70 mg loading, then 50 mg daily
Anidulafungin	Oral 200 mg loading, then 100 mg daily
Caspofungin	Oral 1 gm daily
Fluconazole	Oral or IV 200 mg every 8 h for 6 doses (48 h) loading, then
Flucytosine	200 mg daily
Isavuconazole	IV 100 mg daily
Micafungin	Oral tablet 300 mg every 12 h loading for two doses,
Posaconazole	Then 300 mg daily
Voriconazole	Oral 200 mg every 12 h

peritonitis, the patients should be instructed to avoid oral phosphate binders like calcium carbonate or acetate, sevelamer carbonate [21], and lanthanum carbonate [22] and aluminum containing antacids [23] as they interfere with absorption of fluoroquinolones, lowering their peak concentrations.

The stability of antibiotics in the PD fluid gives an attractive option of premixing of antibiotics by nurses in the PD unit. This reduces the risk of contamination while the patient or caregiver adds the antibiotics for IP antibiotic delivery. The compatibility of antibiotics and their stability in the PD fluids is an important factor influencing treatment success [24]. Cefazolin remains stable for up to 8 days at room temperature and for 14 days if refrigerated in dextrose-based PD solutions and for 7 days at room temperature and for 14 days if refrigerated in Icodextrin [25], with compatibility unaltered if heparin is added [26]. Gentamicin remains stable for 14 days in both dextrose-based PD solutions and Icodextrin both at room temperature and if refrigerated. The stability is reduced by addition of heparin [25, 27]. Ceftazidime in dextrose-based PD solutions remains stable for 4 days at room temperature or 7 days if refrigerated, and in Icodextrin, it remains stable for 2 days at room temperature and for 14 days if refrigerated [25]. Cefepime remains stable for 14 days in dextrose-based PD solutions if refrigerated [28]. Vancomycin remains stable in dextrose-based PD solutions for 28 days at room temperature, with higher ambient temperatures reducing its stability [27]. Vancomycin remains stable in Icodextrin for 14 days till 25 °C [25]. Piperacillin/tazobactam combination therapy is stable for 7 days when refrigerated in dextrose-based PD solutions and in Icodextrin, even with heparin [29]. Table 5.3 summarizes the stability of IP antibiotics [15]. Since the antibiotics are combined in the PD fluid, the compatibility of the antibiotics must be ascertained before they are mixed in the same bag for IP instillation. The most commonly used combination of antibiotics, ceftazidime with cefazolin or vancomycin, or aminoglycosides with cefazolin or vancomycin raised no concern [24, 25]. The incompatibility of aminoglycosides and penicillins does not allow them to be added to the same PD fluid bag [26].

Table 5.3 Duration of antibiotic therapy

Organism	Duration of antibiotic therapy
Coagulase negative staphylococci (*S. epidermidis, S. haemolyticus)*	14 days
Streptococcus viridans	14 days
Corynebacterium species	14 days
Pasteurella multocida	14 days
Staphylococcus aureus	21 days
Enterococcus species	21 days
Pseudomonas species	21 days
Acinetobacter species	21 days
Stenotrophomonas species	21 days
Enteric gram-negative bacteria	21 days

5.3 Special Considerations in Patients on Automated Peritoneal Dialysis

The antibiotic dosing suggested for patients on continuous ambulatory peritoneal dialysis (CAPD) cannot be easily extrapolated to patients on automated peritoneal dialysis (APD). The peritoneal antibiotic clearance may be higher in patients on APD. The shorter antibiotic half-lives during the cycler exchanges decrease the serum and dialysate drug concentrations with the potential of underdosing and inadequate treatment. This is especially for antibiotics with the property of time-dependent killing. In order to be effective, sufficient dwell time is needed to allow or drug absorption. The dosing strategy must allow the antibiotic concentrations to exceed the MIC for at least 50% of treatment time. Vancomycin needs a minimum dwell time of 4 h [30], though 6 h may be better [31] to achieve adequate peritoneal concentration.

In many units, the routine practice is transient conversion to CAPD to ensure adequate antibiotic dosing. While not always easy to implement, at least when using antibiotics that require continuous dosing, this may be a necessary option to resort to.

5.4 Additional Treatment to Be Instituted

Prevention of fungal prophylaxis is done using either oral Nystatin 500,000 U (5 ml of 100,000 Uml) every 6 h or oral fluconazole 100 mg (or 200 mg) once daily for duration of antibiotic therapy peritonitis treatment, to be continued for a subsequent week. The absorption of Icodextrin is less than that of dextrose from the instilled PD fluid dwell. Hence, if the patient is in fluids overload, using Icodextrin may be preferable to treat the fluid overload. Conversely, hypertonic dextrose fluid could be used with shorter dwell times. The use of hypertonic dextrose fluid worsens glycemic control in diabetic patients, and the patients need to be monitored for hyperglycemia and treated appropriately. 500 units per liter of heparin is added if the PD fluid is cloudy to prevent fibrinous occlusion of the catheter lumen. Protein loss in the PD fluid is increased in peritonitis and special attention to nutrition is required in these patients to avoid malnutrition.

5.5 Subsequent Treatment

Is it expected that the majority of PD peritonitis will improve within 48 h of starting antibiotics. Patients are taught to look for visible clearing of PD fluid. On initiation of antimicrobial therapy, three responses are possible: *early response* (normalization of PD fluid WBC count by day 5), *delayed response* (decline in the total WBC count, but remains >100/μl by day 5), and *treatment failure* (non-resolution of PD peritonitis despite 5 days of appropriate antibiotic therapy, temporary or permanent switch to hemodialysis or death) [32]. In up to 20%, there may be a delayed response without necessitating PD catheter removal, with improvement in PD fluid total WBC count by day 5 [32].

On review at 48 h, patient's catheter and exit site are reexamined to look for any tell-tale signs of exit site or tunnel infection. Repeat PD fluid counts are sent and if there is no improvement, repeat cultures are sent as well. The PD fluid total WBC count at 72 h in important for prognostication. PD fluid WBC count >1000/μl [33] or > 1090/μl [34] at 72 h is associated with a high likelihood of failure of treatment.

Depending on the organism grown on culture and its sensitivity, the antibiotic therapy is modified. The duration of commonly used antibiotic therapy is listed in Table 5.3. If the patient is deteriorating clinically, early PD catheter removal may be beneficial to prevent mortality and increased morbidity [15]. If the PD peritonitis does to resolve after 5 days of appropriate therapy, the peritonitis is considered *refractory*. Surgical removal of the PD catheter is recommended at this point. A clinical tweak in therapy that could be implemented in patients with culture negative PD peritonitis whose PD fluid WBC count remains elevated after 5 days of empiric therapy is to upgrade the antibiotics by day 3 or 5 and start the 5 day countdown from that new date. If there is improvement in the PD fluid WBC count, though without normalization, one may continue antibiotics with close observation instead of prompt removal after day 5 [15].

Prolonged antibiotics therapy in refractory peritonitis without timely catheter removal increases the risk of mortality, development of fungal peritonitis, and permanent damage to the peritoneal membrane and prolongs hospital stay [35, 36].

5.6 Treatment of Specific Infections

The duration of antibiotic therapy for each bacterial PD peritonitis is listed in Table 5.3.

5.6.1 Coagulase: Negative Staphylococci

The most common organism causing coagulase negative staphylococcal PD peritonitis are *S. epidermidis* and, less commonly, *S. haemolyticus*. Among staphylococci, these organisms cause infections more commonly than *S. aureus,* despite the latter having greater virulence because host fibrinogen antimicrobial defenses are effective against *S. aureus* but not against coagulase negative staphylococci [37]. Two weeks of IP cefazolin may be sufficient therapy.

After an episode of coagulase negative staphylococcal PD peritonitis, the PD nurse should review the exchange techniques to prevent touch contamination and recurrence of peritonitis [15]. Retraining of the patient and caregiver/s is also advisable. Coagulase negative staphylococcal PD peritonitis has an inherent increased risk of refractory and repeat peritonitis, often a month after successful completion of antibiotic therapy for PD peritonitis [38]. The rate of occurrence of repeat peritonitis is about 12% [39, 40] and is likely secondary to colonization of the PD catheter with a biofilm with presence of mecA and icaAD genes [40]. Repeat peritonitis may require catheter removal. Simultaneous removal and PD catheter reinsertion as a single procedure after the PD fluid WBC count has normalized may be more pragmatic [38].

5.6.2 *Staphylococcus aureus*

PD peritonitis due to *Staphylococcus aureus* usually results from concomitant or prior exit site infection, with or without contributory touch contamination. In methicillin-sensitive *S. aureus* infection, both cefazolin and vancomycin are equally effective [41, 42], and either is given for 3 weeks. In methicillin-resistant *S. aureus* (MRSA) PD peritonitis, IP vancomycin is the treatment of choice [15]. Addition of oral rifampicin for 5 to 7 days may reduce the risk of relapse or repeat *S. aureus* PD peritonitis [41]. If the IP vancomycin in response is insufficient, it may be prudent to consider IP daptomycin, with or without oral rifampicin as salvage therapy [43]. If there is concomitant exit site or catheter tunnel infection, catheter removal may be needed [15]. An important consideration is that Teicoplanin is not a preferred antibiotic in PD peritonitis because the biofilm impairs its MRSA activity [44].

5.6.3 Streptococci

PD peritonitis due to streptococcal infection has a high cure rate of over 85% with 2 weeks of antibiotic therapy being adequate, and most patients are able to continue PD uninterrupted [45, 46]. The *Streptococcus viridans* group (including oralis, sanguis, and gordonii) have a higher risk of relapse [47].

5.6.4 Corynebacteria

Corynebacteria are part of natural skin flora. Antibiotics treatment for 2 weeks is sufficient to treat PD peritonitis caused by Corynebacteria. *Corynebacterium jeikeium* may be resistant to beta-lactamase antibiotics and vancomycin treatment is necessary. Early catheter removal is needed in patients with *Corynebacterium* PD peritonitis and concomitant exit site or tunnel infection.

5.6.5 *Enterococcus*

Enterococcal PD peritonitis is treated with 3 weeks of oral amoxicillin or vancomycin is resistant to cases. Vancomycin use is minimized to prevent vancomycin-resistant enterococci (VRE) emergence. For VRE PD peritonitis, consultation with infectious disease specialists is warranted. Linezolid, either orally or intravenously, and IP daptomycin have been used. Newer drugs like dalbavancin and combination therapy with tigecyline and fosfomycin may be used. IP ampicillin and linezolid lose their bacteriostatic effect on *Enterococcus faecalis* in the presence of PD fluid. Dalbavancin may cause chemical peritonitis when used intraperitoneally [48].

Enterococcal peritonitis as part of polymicrobial injection have poorer outcomes with longer hospital stay, high likelihood of catheter removal, and poor response to therapy with three [49] to four times [50] greater mortality.

5.6.6 *Pseudomonas*

PD peritonitis episodes due to pseudomonas species tend to be severe and less than half are able to affect complete cure [51, 52]. Two sensitive antibiotics are used for treatment for a period of 3 weeks. Early catheter removal, if not responding to 5days of antibiotic treatment, decreases the risk of mortality [51] and increases the likelihood of return to peritoneal dialysis [36, 51]. PD peritonitis due to *Pseudomonas* responded inadequately despite in vitro susceptibility of antibiotics owing to high risk of biofilm production [53].

5.6.7 *Stenotrophomonas maltophilia*

Like *Pseudomonas* PD peritonitis, *Stenotrophomonas* PD peritonitis also requires two drug therapy for 3 week and a combination of trimethoprim–sulfamethoxazole with either a fluoroquinolone like levofloxacin or moxifloxacin, ceftazidime, tigecycline, minocycline or ticarcillin/clavulanic acid is used [54].

5.6.8 *Acinetobacter*

Local susceptibility patterns dictate antibiotic therapy for *Acinetobacter*-induced PD peritonitis. Broad-spectrum cephalosporin, a combination beta-lactam/beta-lactamase inhibitor antibiotic that includes sulbactam or a carbapenem is used for a duration of 3 weeks. A combination of an aminoglycoside and a sulbactam containing antibiotic is used in treatment of carbapenem-resistant *Acinetobacter* PD peritonitis.

5.6.9 Enteric Gram-Negative Bacteria

Enteric gram-negative bacteria (most commonly *Escherichia coli*, *Klebsiella*, and *Enterobacter)* need treatment with antibiotics, based on susceptibility, for a period of 3 weeks. There are higher treatment failure rates and antibiotic resistant than other bacteria [55]. In resistant cases, cefepime (a fourth-generation cephalosporin) or carbapenem should be used.

5.7 Polymicrobial PD Peritonitis

Growth of multiple enteric organisms on culture suggests intra-abdominal pathology due to a surgical cause. These patients need to be evaluated by a surgeon for obstruction, intra-abdominal collection, perforation, etc. Abdominal CT scan may be needed to clinch the diagnosis. The patient may present in an unstable state with hypotension, lactic acidosis, and frank sepsis. There may be elevated levels of amylase in the effluent [56]. The antibiotics chosen need to cover for gram-negative, gram-positive, and anaerobic bacteria. Combination therapy with vancomycin, ceftazidime (or amikacin), and metronidazole is a good option. Alternatively, monotherapy with a carbapenem or piperacillin/tazobactam may be used. After surgical consultation, if laparotomy is need, the PD catheter should be removed, and the antibiotics are continued intravenously.

On the other hand, polymicrobial gram-positive PD peritonitis has a better prognosis with the natural histology being similar to that of a single gram-positive organism. Touch contamination is a possibility and history for the same must be sought. Treatment required is usually antibiotics alone without PD catheter removal [57]. Polymicrobial PD peritonitis is treated with antibiotic therapy for 3 weeks [15].

5.8 Culture Negative Peritonitis

In several instances, the PD fluid cultures remain sterile on repeated cultures. Improper culture techniques of recent antibiotic use are risk factors for culture negative peritonitis [58, 59]. When culture is negative on day 3, repeat WBC count—total and differential, cultures including fungal culture and mycobacterial cultures are sent [15]. If the fluid count normalizes promptly with antibiotics, the organism is preserved to be coagulase-negative *Staphylococcus*, and the recommended treatment is for 2 weeks [15]. However, in several instances, the culture-negative peritonitis is unlikely to be due to gram-positive organism alone, and 3 weeks of combined gram-positive and gram-negative antibiotic therapy is probably beneficial. In about 10% of all culture-negative PD peritonitis, PD catheter removal is necessary [58, 60].

5.9 Fungal PD Peritonitis

PD peritonitis due to fungal infection is a dreaded consequence of doing peritoneal dialysis. Despite prompt PD catheter removal, the risk of mortality and treatment failure remains high [61, 62]. The gram stain sent on the initial PD fluid sample often gives a clue to the diagnosis and allows for prompt initiation of therapy.

The most common fungal pathogenies are *Candida albicans* and *Candida parapsilosis*, the latter being encountered more often [63]. *Candida albicans* PD peritonitis is treated with fluconazole, while other Candida requires an IV echinocandin (caspofungin, anidulafungin, or micafungin) or oral voriconazole [64, 65]. Oral voriconazole is preferred over IV voriconazole because the vehicle cyclodextrin used in IV voriconazole tends to accumulate in patients with ESKD. Oral voriconazole also delivers excellent peritoneal concentration [66].

PD peritonitis due to *Aspergillus* species require treatment with IV amphotericin B or an azole like voriconazole or posaconazole [67]. PD peritonitis due to mucor species or other fungal species, require appropriate anti-fungal treatment.

The mortality from fungal PD peritonitis ranges from 50% [68] to over 90% [69] if the PD catheter is not removed. Hence, prompt catheter removal is advised [15]. Prompt catheter removal lowers the risk of mortality and increases the possibility of resuming PD in the future [62, 68].

The optimal duration of antifungal therapy remains unknown but 2 to 4 weeks after catheter removal seems optimal [69].

5.10 Tuberculous PD Peritonitis

PD peritonitis due to *Mycobacterium tuberculosis* often mimics bacterial peritonitis. The initial PD fluid WBC differential count also may show polymorphonuclear cell predominance in nearly 80% of cases [70–72]. Some clues to the diagnosis may be the presence of fever in over 80% of patients in additional to abdominal pain in 90% of patients [70]. Mycobacterial cultures take long to show growth of organism, and this may delay the diagnosis by over 6 weeks [73]. PD fluid adenosine deaminase and gene XPERT polymerase chain reaction may be used [72, 74], but the former's lack of specificity and the latter's lack of sensitivity make them infective tests to exclude tuberculous (Table 5.4).

Anti-tubercular therapy is as per routine clinical use—a multidrug therapy protocol is used with four drugs for 2 months (typically isoniazid, rifampicin, pyrazinamide, and ethambutol) and two drugs (isoniazid and rifampicin) for 10 months. Patients' response to be monitored for side effects of anti-tubercular therapy. Routine co-administration of pyridoxine is done to prevent isoniazid-induced peripheral neuropathy.

Removal of the PD catheter may not be required in most instances. However, commonly, the catheter may be removed as part of treating resistant "culture negative" PD peritonitis before the mycobacterial cultures grow the organism. Removal of catheter does not translate to a better likelihood of survival [72], the only impacting factor being time of initiation of therapy—earlier the better.

Table 5.4 Drug dosing in tuberculous PD peritonitis (modified) [15]

Drug	Oral dosing
Isoniazid	5 mg/kg daily (maximum dose 300 mg daily) [75]
Rifampicin	450 mg daily for body weight < 50 kg; 600 mg daily for body weight > 50 kg
Pyrazinamide	30 mg/kg three times weekly
Levofloxacin	250 mg every 48 h
Ofloxacin	Oral 200 mg daily [70]
Ethambutol	15 mg/kg every 48 h [75]
Moxifloxacin	Oral 400 mg daily [76, 77]

5.11 Non-tuberculous Mycobacterial (NTM) PD Peritonitis

The diagnosis of non-tuberculous PD peritonitis is often delayed. In culture-negative PD peritonitis or if there is any suspicion of NTM peritonitis, Ziehl–Neelsen staining for acid-fact bacilli is recommended [15]. The delay in diagnosis may range from 6 days to a month [78, 79]. The most common NTM PD peritonitis-causing organisms are *Mycobacterium fortuitum* and *Mycobacterium chelonae* [78, 80, 81]. If the gram stain appears to suggest *Corynebacterium diphtheria*, it is recommended to do a Ziehl–Neelsen stain to look for NTM PD peritonitis [15]. Culture-negative PD peritonitis with persistent peritonitis-related symptoms with concomitant exit site infection is suspicious for the presence of NTM PD peritonitis. The laboratory should prolong incubation of the PF fluid culture to 7 days in addition to doing mycobacterial cultures [79]. The optimum treatment duration is unknown, but a minimum of 6 weeks is suggested [82]. Consultations with infectious disease specialists may be helpful in selecting appropriate anti-mycobacterial therapy. PD catheter removal is also necessary as part of therapy to remove the source of infection [15]. Less than one-fifth of patients with NTM PD peritonitis are able to be restarted on PD. [83]

5.12 Relapsing, Recurrent, and Repeat PD Peritonitis

Relapsing PD peritonitis is one that occurs within 4 weeks of completion of treatment of a prior episode with either the same organism, or a culture-negative PD peritonitis. A culture-positive PD peritonitis episode within 4 weeks of completion of treatment of a culture negative PD peritonitis is also considered to be relapsing. *Recurrent* PD peritonitis is one that occurs within 4 weeks of completion of treatment of a prior episode with a different organism. *Repeat* PD peritonitis is one that occurs more than 4 weeks after completion of treatment of a prior episode with the same organism.

In all three conditions, it may be prudent to consider PD catheter removal. Relapsing peritonitis episodes are associated with a lower likelihood of cure, decrease in ultrafiltration, and increase risk of technique failure [84]. Recurrent PD peritonitis has a poorer prognosis than relapsing PD peritonitis [84, 85]. It has been observed that centers with larger PD programs have lower rates of relapsing and recurrent peritonitis [60]. Prolonged antibiotic use in these patients increases the risk of secondary fungal PD peritonitis [86].

5.13 Conclusions

PD peritonitis may be caused by a variety of organisms—bacterial, fungal, or mycobacterial. Early diagnosis and prompt initiation of therapy, with or without timely catheter removal (as indicated), are the mainstays of treatment in order to effect cure.

5.14 Important Points

- Empiric antimicrobial therapy must be initiated as soon as possible after samples are collected for PF fluid counts, gram stain, and cultures.
- Antibiotics may need to be changed based on susceptibility pattern on culture sensitivity reports.
- Duration of therapy depends on identification of organism on culture.
- Empiric antifungal therapy is needed for all patients on initiating antibiotic therapy.
- If PD peritonitis persists despite 5 days of appropriate therapy, it is deemed refractory and the PD catheter needs to be removed.
- Fungal PD peritonitis requires prompt PD catheter removal.
- Tubercular and non-tubercular mycobacterial PD peritonitis needs high index of suspicion and prolonged mycobacterial culture of PD fluid.

References

1. Teitelbaum I. Cloudy Peritoneal Dialysate: It's not Always Infection. In: Ronco C, Dell'Aquila R, Rodighiero MP, eds. Contributions to nephrology. KARGER; 2006:187–194. https://doi.org/10.1159/000093594.
2. Chow KM, Chow VCY, Szeto CC, Law MC, Leung CB, Li PKT. Continuous ambulatory peritoneal dialysis peritonitis: broth inoculation culture versus water lysis method. Nephron Clin Pract. 2007;105(3):c121–5. https://doi.org/10.1159/000098643.
3. Tanratananon D, Deekae S, Raksasuk S, Srithongkul T. Evaluation of different methods to improve culture-negative peritoneal dialysis-related peritonitis: a single-center study. Ann Med Surg. 2012;2021(63):102139. https://doi.org/10.1016/j.amsu.2021.01.087.
4. Lee CC, Sun CY, Chang KC, Wu MS. Positive dialysate gram stain predicts outcome of empirical antibiotic therapy for peritoneal dialysis-associated peritonitis. Ther Apher Dial. 2010;14(2):201–8. https://doi.org/10.1111/j.1744-9987.2009.00784.x.
5. Buchanan R, Fan S, NicFhogartaigh C. Performance of gram stains and 3 culture methods in the analysis of peritoneal dialysis fluid. Perit Dial Int J Int Soc Perit Dial. 2019;39(2):190–2. https://doi.org/10.3747/pdi.2018.00087.
6. de Fijter CWH. Gram stain of peritoneal dialysis fluid: the potential of direct policy-determining importance in early diagnosis of fungal peritonitis. Perit Dial Int J Int Soc Perit Dial. 2019;39(6):574–5. https://doi.org/10.3747/pdi.2019.00073.
7. Kanjanabuch T, Puapatanakul P, Saejew T, et al. The culture from peritoneal dialysis catheter enhances yield of microorganism identification in peritoneal dialysis-related peritonitis. Perit Dial Int J Int Soc Perit Dial. 2020;40(1):93–5. https://doi.org/10.1177/0896860819878387.
8. Galvao C, Swartz R, Rocher L, Reynolds J, Starmann B, Wilson D. Acinetobacter peritonitis during chronic peritoneal dialysis. Am J Kidney Dis Off J Natl Kidney Found. 1989;14(2):101–4. https://doi.org/10.1016/s0272-6386(89)80184-2.
9. Mugambi SM, Ullian ME. Bacteremia, sepsis, and peritonitis with Pasteurella multocida in a peritoneal dialysis patient. Perit Dial Int J Int Soc Perit Dial. 2010;30(3):381–3. https://doi.org/10.3747/pdi.2009.00186.
10. Morduchowicz G, van Dyk DJ, Wittenberg C, Winkler J, Boner G. Bacteremia complicating peritonitis in peritoneal dialysis patients. Am J Nephrol. 1993;13(4):278–80. https://doi.org/10.1159/000168634.

11. Penven M, Lalieu A, Boruchowicz A, et al. Bacteremia caused by Elizabethkingia miricola in a patient with acute pancreatitis and peritoneal dialysis. Médecine Mal Infect. 2020;50(4):379–81. https://doi.org/10.1016/j.medmal.2020.01.009.
12. Flanigan MJ, Freeman RM, Lim VS. Cellular response to peritonitis among peritoneal dialysis patients. Am J Kidney Dis Off J Natl Kidney Found. 1985;6(6):420–4. https://doi.org/10.1016/s0272-6386(85)80105-0.
13. Muthucumarana K, Howson P, Crawford D, Burrows S, Swaminathan R, Irish A. The relationship between presentation and the time of initial Administration of Antibiotics with Outcomes of peritonitis in peritoneal dialysis patients: the PROMPT study. Kidney Int Rep. 2016;1(2):65–72. https://doi.org/10.1016/j.ekir.2016.05.003.
14. Oki R, Tsuji S, Hamasaki Y, et al. Time until treatment initiation is associated with catheter survival in peritoneal dialysis-related peritonitis. Sci Rep. 2021;11(1):6547. https://doi.org/10.1038/s41598-021-86071-y.
15. Li PKT, Chow KM, Cho Y, et al. ISPD peritonitis guideline recommendations: 2022 update on prevention and treatment. Perit Dial Int J Int Soc Perit Dial. 2022;42(2):110–53. https://doi.org/10.1177/08968608221080586.
16. Zelenitsky SA, Howarth J, Lagacé-Wiens P, et al. Microbiological trends and antimicrobial resistance in peritoneal dialysis-related peritonitis, 2005 to 2014. Perit Dial Int J Int Soc Perit Dial. 2017;37(2):170–6. https://doi.org/10.3747/pdi.2016.00136.
17. Lui SL, Cheng SW, Ng F, et al. Cefazolin plus netilmicin versus cefazolin plus ceftazidime for treating CAPD peritonitis: effect on residual renal function. Kidney Int. 2005;68(5):2375–80. https://doi.org/10.1111/j.1523-1755.2005.00700.x.
18. Tokgoz B, Somdas MA, Ucar C, et al. Correlation between hearing loss and peritonitis frequency and administration of ototoxic intraperitoneal antibiotics in patients with CAPD. Ren Fail. 2010;32(2):179–84. https://doi.org/10.3109/08860220903491224.
19. Lortholary O, Tod M, Cohen Y, Petitjean O. Aminoglycosides. Med Clin North Am. 1995;79(4):761–87. https://doi.org/10.1016/s0025-7125(16)30038-4.
20. Kitrungphaiboon T, Puapatanakul P, Chuengsaman P, et al. Intraperitoneal Cefepime monotherapy versus combination therapy of cefazolin plus ceftazidime for empirical treatment of CAPD-associated peritonitis: a multicenter, open-label, noninferiority, randomized, controlled trial. Am J Kidney Dis Off J Natl Kidney Found. 2019;74(5):601–9. https://doi.org/10.1053/j.ajkd.2019.05.011.
21. Kays MB, Overholser BR, Mueller BA, Moe SM, Sowinski KM. Effects of sevelamer hydrochloride and calcium acetate on the oral bioavailability of ciprofloxacin. Am J Kidney Dis Off J Natl Kidney Found. 2003;42(6):1253–9. https://doi.org/10.1053/j.ajkd.2003.08.027.
22. How PP, Fischer JH, Arruda JA, Lau AH. Effects of lanthanum carbonate on the absorption and oral bioavailability of ciprofloxacin. Clin J Am Soc Nephrol CJASN. 2007;2(6):1235–40. https://doi.org/10.2215/CJN.01580407.
23. Golper TA, Hartstein AI, Morthland VH, Christensen JM. Effects of antacids and dialysate dwell times on multiple-dose pharmacokinetics of oral ciprofloxacin in patients on continuous ambulatory peritoneal dialysis. Antimicrob Agents Chemother. 1987;31(11):1787–90. https://doi.org/10.1128/AAC.31.11.1787.
24. So SWY, Chen L, Woo AYH, et al. Stability and compatibility of antibiotics in peritoneal dialysis solutions. Clin Kidney J. 2022;15(6):1071–8. https://doi.org/10.1093/ckj/sfac012.
25. Ranganathan D, Naicker S, Wallis SC, Lipman J, Ratanjee SK, Roberts JA. Stability of antibiotics for intraperitoneal Administration in Extraneal 7.5% Icodextrin peritoneal dialysis bags (STAB study). Perit Dial Int J Int Soc Perit Dial. 2016;36(4):421–6. https://doi.org/10.3747/pdi.2015.00062.
26. de Vin F, Rutherford P, Faict D. Intraperitoneal administration of drugs in peritoneal dialysis patients: a review of compatibility and guidance for clinical use. Perit Dial Int J Int Soc Perit Dial. 2009;29(1):5–15.
27. Dooley DP, Tyler JR, Wortham WG, et al. Prolonged stability of antimicrobial activity in peritoneal dialysis solutions. Perit Dial Int J Int Soc Perit Dial. 2003;23(1):58–62.

28. Williamson JC, Volles DF, Lynch PL, Rogers PD, Haverstick DM. Stability of cefepime in peritoneal dialysis solution. Ann Pharmacother. 1999;33(9):906–9. https://doi.org/10.1345/aph.18336.
29. Mendes K, Harmanjeet H, Sedeeq M, et al. Stability of Meropenem and piperacillin/Tazobactam with heparin in various peritoneal dialysis solutions. Perit Dial Int J Int Soc Perit Dial. 2018;38(6):430–40. https://doi.org/10.3747/pdi.2017.00274.
30. Fish R, Nipah R, Jones C, Finney H, Fan SLS. Intraperitoneal vancomycin concentrations during peritoneal dialysis-associated peritonitis: correlation with serum levels. Perit Dial Int J Int Soc Perit Dial. 2012;32(3):332–8. https://doi.org/10.3747/pdi.2010.00294.
31. Falbo Dos Reis P, Barretti P, Marinho L, Balbi AL, Awdishu L, Ponce D. Pharmacokinetics of intraperitoneal vancomycin and amikacin in automated peritoneal dialysis patients with peritonitis. Front Pharmacol. 2021;12:658014. https://doi.org/10.3389/fphar.2021.658014.
32. Tantiyavarong P, Traitanon O, Chuengsaman P, Patumanond J, Tasanarong A. Dialysate white blood cell change after initial antibiotic treatment represented the patterns of response in peritoneal dialysis-related peritonitis. Int J Nephrol. 2016;2016:6217135. https://doi.org/10.1155/2016/6217135.
33. Nochaiwong S, Ruengorn C, Koyratkoson K, et al. A clinical risk prediction tool for peritonitis-associated treatment failure in peritoneal dialysis patients. Sci Rep. 2018;8(1):14797. https://doi.org/10.1038/s41598-018-33196-2.
34. Chow KM, Szeto CC, Cheung KKT, et al. Predictive value of dialysate cell counts in peritonitis complicating peritoneal dialysis. Clin J Am Soc Nephrol CJASN. 2006;1(4):768–73. https://doi.org/10.2215/CJN.01010306.
35. Choi P, Nemati E, Banerjee A, Preston E, Levy J, Brown E. Peritoneal dialysis catheter removal for acute peritonitis: a retrospective analysis of factors associated with catheter removal and prolonged postoperative hospitalization. Am J Kidney Dis Off J Natl Kidney Found. 2004;43(1):103–11. https://doi.org/10.1053/j.ajkd.2003.08.046.
36. Lu W, Kwan BCH, Chow KM, et al. Peritoneal dialysis-related peritonitis caused by pseudomonas species: insight from a post-millennial case series. PLoS One. 2018;13(5):e0196499. https://doi.org/10.1371/journal.pone.0196499.
37. Prasad JM, Negrón O, Du X, et al. Host fibrinogen drives antimicrobial function in Staphylococcus aureus peritonitis through bacterial-mediated prothrombin activation. Proc Natl Acad Sci U S A. 2021;118(1):e2009837118. https://doi.org/10.1073/pnas.2009837118.
38. Mitra A, Teitelbaum I. Is it safe to simultaneously remove and replace infected peritoneal dialysis catheters? Review of the literature and suggested guidelines. Adv Perit Dial Conf Perit Dial. 2003;19:255–9.
39. Szeto CC, Kwan BCH, Chow KM, et al. Coagulase negative staphylococcal peritonitis in peritoneal dialysis patients: review of 232 consecutive cases. Clin J Am Soc Nephrol CJASN. 2008;3(1):91–7. https://doi.org/10.2215/CJN.03070707.
40. Camargo CH, Cunha M de LR de S da, Caramori JCT, Mondelli AL, Montelli AC, Barretti P. Peritoneal dialysis-related peritonitis due to coagulase-negative staphylococcus: a review of 115 cases in a Brazilian center. Clin J Am Soc Nephrol CJASN. 2014;9(6):1074–81. https://doi.org/10.2215/CJN.09280913.
41. Szeto CC, Chow KM, Kwan BCH, et al. Staphylococcus aureus peritonitis complicates peritoneal dialysis: review of 245 consecutive cases. Clin J Am Soc Nephrol CJASN. 2007;2(2):245–51. https://doi.org/10.2215/CJN.03180906.
42. Govindarajulu S, Hawley CM, McDonald SP, et al. Staphylococcus aureus peritonitis in Australian peritoneal dialysis patients: predictors, treatment, and outcomes in 503 cases. Perit Dial Int J Int Soc Perit Dial. 2010;30(3):311–9. https://doi.org/10.3747/pdi.2008.00258.
43. Lin SY, Ho MW, Liu JH, et al. Successful salvage of peritoneal catheter in unresolved methicillin-resistant staphylococcus aureus peritonitis by combination treatment with daptomycin and rifampin. Blood Purif. 2011;32(4):249–52. https://doi.org/10.1159/000328028.
44. Tobudic S, Kern S, Kussmann M, Forstner C, Burgmann H. Effect of peritoneal dialysis fluids on activity of Teicoplanin against methicillin-resistant Staphylococcus aureus biofilm. Perit Dial Int J Int Soc Perit Dial. 2019;39(3):293–4. https://doi.org/10.3747/pdi.2018.00168.

45. O'Shea S, Hawley CM, McDonald SP, et al. Streptococcal peritonitis in Australian peritoneal dialysis patients: predictors, treatment and outcomes in 287 cases. BMC Nephrol. 2009;10:19. https://doi.org/10.1186/1471-2369-10-19.
46. Santos JE, Rodríguez Magariños C, García Gago L, et al. Long-term trends in the incidence of peritoneal dialysis-related peritonitis disclose an increasing relevance of streptococcal infections: a longitudinal study. PLoS One. 2020;15(12):e0244283. https://doi.org/10.1371/journal.pone.0244283.
47. Chao CT, Lee SY, Yang WS, et al. Viridans streptococci in peritoneal dialysis peritonitis: clinical courses and long-term outcomes. Perit Dial Int J Int Soc Perit Dial. 2015;35(3):333–41. https://doi.org/10.3747/pdi.2013.00108.
48. Van Matre ET, Teitelbaum I, Kiser TH. Intravenous and intraperitoneal pharmacokinetics of Dalbavancin in peritoneal dialysis patients. Antimicrob Agents Chemother. 2020;64(5):e02089–19. https://doi.org/10.1128/AAC.02089-19.
49. Edey M, Hawley CM, McDonald SP, et al. Enterococcal peritonitis in Australian peritoneal dialysis patients: predictors, treatment and outcomes in 116 cases. Nephrol Dial Transplant Off Publ Eur Dial Transpl Assoc–Eur Ren Assoc. 2010;25(4):1272–8. https://doi.org/10.1093/ndt/gfp641.
50. Szeto CC, Ng JKC, Chow KM, et al. Treatment of Enterococcal peritonitis in peritoneal dialysis patients by Oral amoxicillin or intra-peritoneal Vancomcyin: a retrospective study. Kidney Blood Press Res. 2017;42(5):837–43. https://doi.org/10.1159/000484426.
51. Siva B, Hawley CM, McDonald SP, et al. Pseudomonas peritonitis in Australia: predictors, treatment, and outcomes in 191 cases. Clin J Am Soc Nephrol CJASN. 2009;4(5):957–64. https://doi.org/10.2215/CJN.00010109.
52. Szeto CC, Chow KM, Leung CB, et al. Clinical course of peritonitis due to pseudomonas species complicating peritoneal dialysis: a review of 104 cases. Kidney Int. 2001;59(6):2309–15. https://doi.org/10.1046/j.1523-1755.2001.00748.x.
53. Dos Santos ACML, Hernandes RT, Montelli AC, et al. Clinical and microbiological factors predicting outcomes of nonfermenting gram-negative bacilli peritonitis in peritoneal dialysis. Sci Rep. 2021;11(1):12248. https://doi.org/10.1038/s41598-021-91410-0.
54. Abbott IJ, Peleg AY. Stenotrophomonas, Achromobacter, and nonmelioid Burkholderia species: antimicrobial resistance and therapeutic strategies. Semin Respir Crit Care Med. 2015;36(1):99–110. https://doi.org/10.1055/s-0034-1396929.
55. Wu H, Yi C, Zhang D, et al. Changes of antibiotic resistance over time among *Escherichia coli* peritonitis in southern China. Perit Dial Int J Int Soc Perit Dial. 2022;42(2):218–22. https://doi.org/10.1177/08968608211045272.
56. Harwell CM, Newman LN, Cacho CP, Mulligan DC, Schulak JA, Friedlander MA. Abdominal catastrophe: visceral injury as a cause of peritonitis in patients treated by peritoneal dialysis. Perit Dial Int J Int Soc Perit Dial. 1997;17(6):586–94.
57. Szeto CC, Chow KM, Wong TYH, Leung CB, Li PKT. Conservative management of polymicrobial peritonitis complicating peritoneal dialysis–a series of 140 consecutive cases. Am J Med. 2002;113(9):728–33. https://doi.org/10.1016/s0002-9343(02)01364-5.
58. Szeto CC, Wong TYH, Chow KM, Leung CB, Li PKT. The clinical course of culture-negative peritonitis complicating peritoneal dialysis. Am J Kidney Dis Off J Natl Kidney Found. 2003;42(3):567–74. https://doi.org/10.1016/s0272-6386(03)00790-x.
59. Fahim M, Hawley CM, McDonald SP, et al. Culture-negative peritonitis in peritoneal dialysis patients in Australia: predictors, treatment, and outcomes in 435 cases. Am J Kidney Dis Off J Natl Kidney Found. 2010;55(4):690–7. https://doi.org/10.1053/j.ajkd.2009.11.015.
60. Htay H, Cho Y, Pascoe EM, et al. Multicentre registry data analysis comparing outcomes of culture-negative peritonitis and different subtypes of culture-positive peritonitis in peritoneal dialysis patients. Perit Dial Int J Int Soc Perit Dial. 2020;40(1):47–56. https://doi.org/10.1177/0896860819879891.
61. Nadeau-Fredette AC, Bargman JM. Characteristics and outcomes of fungal peritonitis in a modern north American cohort. Perit Dial Int J Int Soc Perit Dial. 2015;35(1):78–84. https://doi.org/10.3747/pdi.2013.00179.

62. Chang TI, Kim HW, Park JT, et al. Early catheter removal improves patient survival in peritoneal dialysis patients with fungal peritonitis: results of ninety-four episodes of fungal peritonitis at a single center. Perit Dial Int J Int Soc Perit Dial. 2011;31(1):60–6. https://doi.org/10.3747/pdi.2009.00057.
63. Auricchio S, Giovenzana ME, Pozzi M, et al. Fungal peritonitis in peritoneal dialysis: a 34-year single Centre evaluation. Clin Kidney J. 2018;11(6):874–80. https://doi.org/10.1093/ckj/sfy045.
64. Matuszkiewicz-Rowinska J. Update on fungal peritonitis and its treatment. Perit Dial Int J Int Soc Perit Dial. 2009;29(Suppl 2):S161–5.
65. Giacobino J, Montelli AC, Barretti P, et al. Fungal peritonitis in patients undergoing peritoneal dialysis (PD) in Brazil: molecular identification, biofilm production and antifungal susceptibility of the agents. Med Mycol. 2016;54(7):725–32. https://doi.org/10.1093/mmy/myw030.
66. Peng LW, Lien YHH. Pharmacokinetics of single, oral-dose voriconazole in peritoneal dialysis patients. Am J Kidney Dis Off J Natl Kidney Found. 2005;45(1):162–6. https://doi.org/10.1053/j.ajkd.2004.09.017.
67. Dotis J, Kondou A, Koukloumperi E, et al. Aspergillus peritonitis in peritoneal dialysis patients: a systematic review. J Mycol Medicale. 2020;30(4):101037. https://doi.org/10.1016/j.mycmed.2020.101037.
68. Goldie SJ, Kiernan-Tridle L, Torres C, et al. Fungal peritonitis in a large chronic peritoneal dialysis population: a report of 55 episodes. Am J Kidney Dis Off J Natl Kidney Found. 1996;28(1):86–91. https://doi.org/10.1016/s0272-6386(96)90135-3.
69. Wang AY, Yu AW, Li PK, et al. Factors predicting outcome of fungal peritonitis in peritoneal dialysis: analysis of a 9-year experience of fungal peritonitis in a single center. Am J Kidney Dis Off J Natl Kidney Found. 2000;36(6):1183–92. https://doi.org/10.1053/ajkd.2000.19833.
70. Akpolat T. Tuberculous peritonitis. Perit Dial Int J Int Soc Perit Dial. 2009;29(Suppl 2):S166–9.
71. Talwani R, Horvath JA. Tuberculous peritonitis in patients undergoing continuous ambulatory peritoneal dialysis: case report and review. Clin Infect Dis Off Publ Infect Dis Soc Am. 2000;31(1):70–5. https://doi.org/10.1086/313919.
72. Thomson BKA, Vaughan S, Momciu B. Mycobacterium tuberculosis peritonitis in peritoneal dialysis patients: a scoping review. Nephrol Carlton Vic. 2022;27(2):133–44. https://doi.org/10.1111/nep.13997.
73. Al Sahlawi M, Bargman JM, Perl J. Peritoneal dialysis-associated peritonitis: suggestions for management and mistakes to avoid. Kidney Med. 2020;2(4):467–75. https://doi.org/10.1016/j.xkme.2020.04.010.
74. Lye WC. Rapid diagnosis of mycobacterium tuberculous peritonitis in two continuous ambulatory peritoneal dialysis patients, using DNA amplification by polymerase chain reaction. Adv Perit Dial Conf Perit Dial. 2002;18:154–7.
75. Unsal A, Ahbap E, Basturk T, et al. Tuberculosis in dialysis patients: a nine-year retrospective analysis. J Infect Dev Ctries. 2013;7(3):208–13. https://doi.org/10.3855/jidc.2664.
76. Xu R, Yang Z, Qu Z, et al. Intraperitoneal vancomycin plus either Oral moxifloxacin or intraperitoneal ceftazidime for the treatment of peritoneal dialysis-related peritonitis: a randomized controlled pilot study. Am J Kidney Dis Off J Natl Kidney Found. 2017;70(1):30–7. https://doi.org/10.1053/j.ajkd.2016.11.008.
77. Skalioti C, Tsaganos T, Stamatiadis D, Giamarellos-Bourboulis EJ, Boletis J, Kanellakopoulou K. Pharmacokinetics of moxifloxacin in patients undergoing continuous ambulatory peritoneal dialysis. Perit Dial Int J Int Soc Perit Dial. 2009;29(5):575–9.
78. Fung WWS, Chow KM, Li PKT, Szeto CC. Clinical course of peritoneal dialysis-related peritonitis due to non-tuberculosis mycobacterium–a single Centre experience spanning 20 years. Perit Dial Int J Int Soc Perit Dial. 2022;42(2):204–11. https://doi.org/10.1177/08968608211042434.
79. Bnaya A, Wiener-Well Y, Soetendorp H, et al. Nontuberculous mycobacteria infections of peritoneal dialysis patients: a multicenter study. Perit Dial Int J Int Soc Perit Dial. 2021;41(3):284–91. https://doi.org/10.1177/0896860820923461.

80. Washida N, Itoh H. The role of non-tuberculous mycobacteria in peritoneal dialysis-related infections: a literature review. Contrib Nephrol. 2018;196:155–61. https://doi.org/10.1159/000485716.
81. Jiang SH, Roberts DM, Clayton PA, Jardine M. Non-tuberculous mycobacterial PD peritonitis in Australia. Int Urol Nephrol. 2013;45(5):1423–8. https://doi.org/10.1007/s11255-012-0328-4.
82. Renaud CJ, Subramanian S, Tambyah PA, Lee EJC. The clinical course of rapidly growing nontuberculous mycobacterial peritoneal dialysis infections in Asians: a case series and literature review. Nephrol Carlton Vic. 2011;16(2):174–9. https://doi.org/10.1111/j.1440-1797.2010.01370.x.
83. Song Y, Wu J, Yan H, Chen J. Peritoneal dialysis-associated nontuberculous mycobacterium peritonitis: a systematic review of reported cases. Nephrol Dial Transplant Off Publ Eur Dial Transpl Assoc–Eur Ren Assoc. 2012;27(4):1639–44. https://doi.org/10.1093/ndt/gfr504.
84. Szeto CC, Kwan BCH, Chow KM, et al. Recurrent and relapsing peritonitis: causative organisms and response to treatment. Am J Kidney Dis Off J Natl Kidney Found. 2009;54(4):702–10. https://doi.org/10.1053/j.ajkd.2009.04.032.
85. Burke M, Hawley CM, Badve SV, et al. Relapsing and recurrent peritoneal dialysis-associated peritonitis: a multicenter registry study. Am J Kidney Dis Off J Natl Kidney Found. 2011;58(3):429–36. https://doi.org/10.1053/j.ajkd.2011.03.022.
86. Szeto CC, Ng JKC, Wing-Shing Fung W, et al. Extended antibiotic therapy for the prevention of relapsing and recurrent peritonitis in peritoneal dialysis patients: a randomized controlled trial. Clin Kidney J. 2021;14(3):991–7. https://doi.org/10.1093/ckj/sfaa256.

Ultrafiltration Failure in PD Peritonitis

6

Tarun Jeloka, Edwin Fernando, and Sudakshina Ghosh

A 43-year-old male with end stage kidney disease (ESKD) was initiated on peritoneal dialysis in July 2011. His other comorbidities included left above-knee amputation following a road traffic accident in the past. He was doing 3 exchanges with 2.5%, 2 liters of dextrose containing fluid, over 24 h. His medications included hematinics, calcium, and erythropoietin. His peritoneal equilibration test (PET) done after 1 month was of low average (Fig. 6.1a) and KT/V was 1.72.

On 15th April 2013, he presented with cloudy effluent, abdominal pain, and fever. He had PD peritonitis and culture grew *Staphylococcus epidermidis*. He responded to intraperitoneal vancomycin. However, he had drop in urine output from 500 ml to 200 ml/day, and his ultrafiltration dropped from 600–700 ml to 300–400 ml/day. He had edema of his feet and legs. He was advised high dose of diuretics. After 2 weeks, he was better and was back to regular prescription with improved urine output and ultrafiltration.

On 27th April 2017, he again had PD peritonitis and culture grew *Burkholderia*, which was treated with intravenous Meropenem. He had drop in UF and required 4.25% dextrose for maintaining euvolemia. His urine output was about 100 ml/day and required 4.25% bag overnight to achieve about 600 ml/day of UF. His repeat PET test revealed transition to high average transport characteristic (Fig. 6.1b).

T. Jeloka (✉)
Department of Nephrology, Manipal Hospitals, Pune, India

E. Fernando
Stanley Hospital, Chennai, India

S. Ghosh
Regency Medical Centre, Dar es Salaam, Tanzania

G. Abraham et al. (eds.), *Diagnosis and Management of Complications of Peritoneal Dialysis related Peritonitis*,
https://doi.org/10.1007/978-981-99-2275-8_6

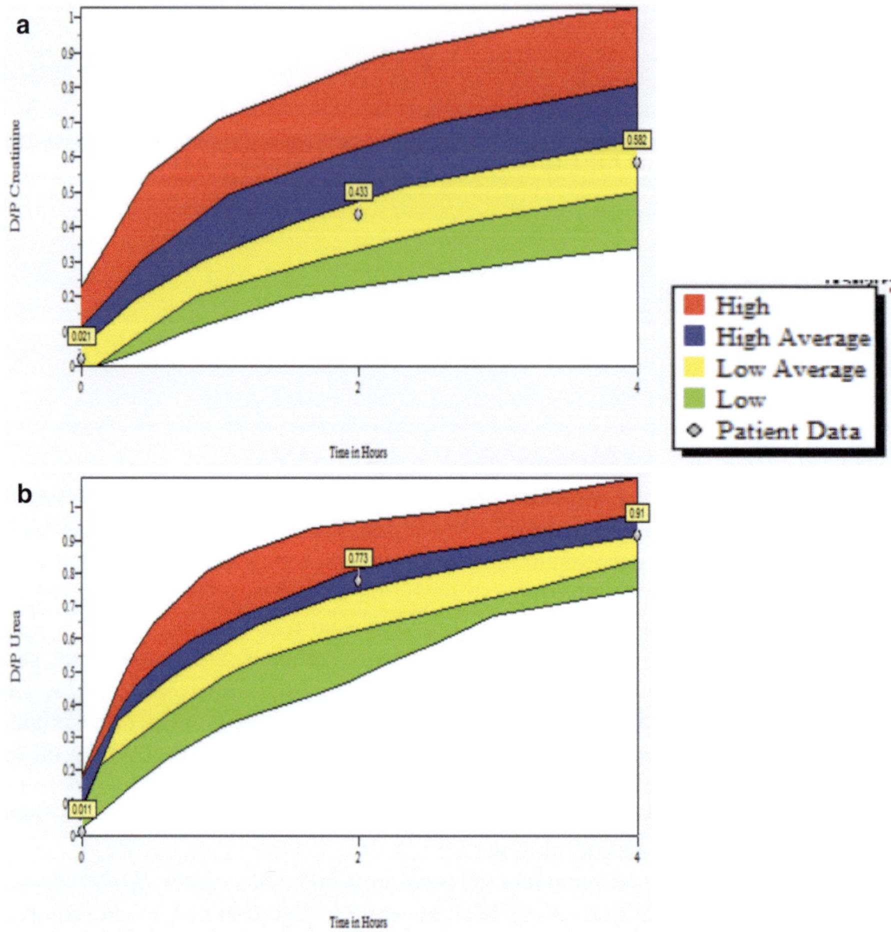

Fig. 6.1 PET characteristic of the patient 1 month after start of dialysis and after episodes of PD peritonitis (6 years after start). (**a**) PET showing low average characteristic in initial part of his dialysis period. (**b**) PET showing transition to high average characteristic after several episodes of pd. peritonitis

He presented with two episodes of pulmonary edema in 2018, which were managed with parenteral diuretics and short frequent exchanges of peritoneal dialysis. He had his third episode of PD peritonitis on 19th July 2019, which was culture negative and was treated with cefepime. After this episode, he became anuric and had an ultrafiltration of only 100–200 ml in 24 h. He also had developed hypertension and required calcium channel blockers for blood pressure control. He was advised to shift to hemodialysis.

This index case highlights the occurrence of ultrafiltration failure (UFF) during an episode of PD peritonitis, which initially was transient and later was permanent.

6.1 Etiology and Pathogenesis

Transcapillary ultrafiltration of water occurs via ultra-small pores (aquaporin 1) and small pores. Ultra-small pores contribute to about 40% of water removal. Peritonitis and consequent inflammation leads to increased permeability of peritoneal vessels. During a peritonitis episode, glucose, the osmotic agent in PD fluid, dissipates faster because of enhanced absorption through these leaky capillaries and reduces the ultrafiltration. In addition, systemic inflammation and certain nephrotoxic drugs used to treat PD peritonitis may reduce the glomerular filtration rate (GFR), leading to clinical evidence of fluid overload [1].

Recurrent PD peritonitis causes structural changes in the peritoneum leading to change in transport characteristics toward "high" transporter status. This again is a long-term effect of peritonitis and is referred as Type 1 UFF. The pathogenesis of this type of UFF includes neo-angiogenesis with leaky capillaries leading to increased effective peritoneal surface area and rapid transport of solutes and reduced UF. This occurs due to prolonged exposure of the peritoneum to glucose, glucose degradation products, and release of proinflammatory and angiogenic mediators in response to recurrent peritonitis (Fig. 6.2a, b).

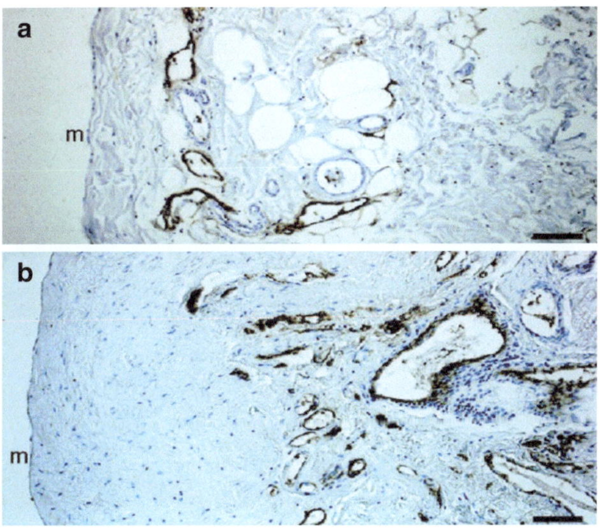

Fig. 6.2 Modifications in peritoneal membrane over 5 years on peritoneal dialysis—loss of mesothelial integrity, submesothelial fibrosis, and vascular proliferation. (**a**) at the beginning of PD; (**b**) after 5 years on PD (acquired from ref. [2])

6.2 Clinical Features

Apart from features of active peritonitis, these patients may have decrease in urine output and ultrafiltration. Patients may complain of swelling of extremities, increasing shortness of breath and increase in weight. There is appearance of edema, raised jugular venous pressure, increased blood pressure, and basal crackles on chest examination.

Depending upon the pathogenesis as described above, UFF may be transient or permanent. Transient UFF occurs during and immediately following an episode of peritonitis. The UF resumes with correction of peritonitis and inflammation. However, with recurrent peritonitis episodes, the UF failure becomes irreversible and leads to fluid overload and possible shift to hemodialysis.

6.3 Diagnosis

Ultrafiltration failure (UFF) can be diagnosed in a patient with clinical evidence of hypervolemia or daily charts showing decrease in UF on consecutive days. Modified peritoneal equilibration test (PET) can document the low UF but is not routinely required for PD peritonitis, as PD records over the previous few days may be helpful in making the diagnosis. Before labeling as UFF due to PD peritonitis, one should first rule out non-adherence, incorrect dialysis prescription, hypoalbuminemia, and mechanical causes like leaks and catheter migration (Fig. 6.3).

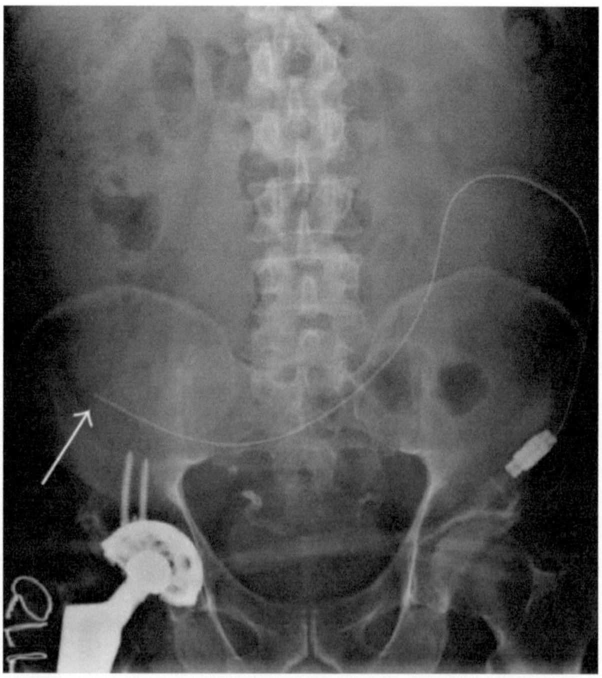

Fig. 6.3 Catheter migration as shown in X ray abdomen

6.4 Differential Diagnosis

Sometimes, there might be adhesion formation as a result of recurrent peritonitis. This may lead to sequestration of fluid within the peritoneal cavity and present as poor ultrafiltration. Identification and possible surgical adhesiolysis may improve this condition. However, occurrence of encapsulating peritoneal sclerosis (EPS), a rare complication of long-term PD, has a relatively poor prognosis, and most cases result in shift to hemodialysis.

True UFF (Table 6.1) occurs in 10–40% of patients with poor UF and is an important cause of technique failure and switch to hemodialysis. True UFF can be diagnosed and characterized by doing a modified "Peritoneal Equilibration test" and looking at "sodium sieving." UFF is diagnosed when ultrafiltration is <400 ml after 4 hours' dwell with 4.25% dextrose containing fluid.

There are four types of UFF—Type 1 as fast transporter status seen usually after a peritonitis episode, Type 2 associated with loss of aquaporins, Type 3 seen in sclerosis or adhesions, and Type 4 with increased lymphatic absorption. The ratio of dialysate to plasma (D/P) creatinine and sodium sieving can be used to differentiate between these types. Management depends on early identification and specific management of cause, if possible (Table 6.1). The outcome of UFF is poor and most patients need shifting to hemodialysis.

Table 6.1 Characteristics of different types of ultrafiltration failure

UFF types	Characteristics	Features	Management	Outcome
Type 1 UFF	Extremely rapid solute transport	Inability to generate ultrafiltration is gradual and permanent	1. Increase concentration of dextrose fluid 2. Automated PD 3. Temporary cessation of PD Remesothelialization (4 weeks / 1 year effect) 4. ACEI / ARBs—Prevent (4 yrs)	? EPS—Switch to HD
Type 2 UFF	Loss of aquaporin function	Cause of functional alteration unknown	Aquaporin 1 upregulated by high dose steroids? Clinical significance	Finally shift to HD
Type 3 UFF	Decreased solute transport related to decreased functional surface area	Secondary to recent episode of PD peritonitis	Early diagnosis and timely switch to HD EPS—surgical enterolysis, immunosuppression, tamoxifen	? EPS Shift to HD
Type 4 UFF	Increased lymphatic and postcapillary absorption—membrane transport function is intact		1. Shorter dwells 2. Higher concentration of dextrose fluid/7.5% icodextrin 3. Avoid larger volume dwells leading to increased intra-abdominal pressure	Poor; shift to HD

6.5 Treatment

Prevention of Type 1 UFF aims at peritonitis prevention and timely and appropriate treatment of PD peritonitis. This includes appropriate exit site care with local antimicrobial prophylaxis and, if infected, treatment of exit site infection with appropriate antibiotic for at least 2 weeks. Early removal of catheter is needed in cases of tunnel infection and fungal or non-responding peritonitis infection. Use of icodextrin or physiological solutions, which are peritoneal membrane friendly, may prevent UFF for a longer period of time. Dietary modifications like salt and fluid restrictions help manage the fluid overload situations.

Transient UFF—use of hypertonic solutions like 4.25% dextrose or icodextrin [3]—may help manage the transient UFF during its acute phase. Decreasing the dwell time and use of automated PD machine also helps manage UFF (Table 6.2).

Permanent UFF—Management of Type 1 UFF is rather challenging and is an important cause of technique failure leading to shift to hemodialysis. Peritoneal resting for more than 4 weeks has shown to decrease the mass transfer coefficients for urea and creatinine and increase in ultrafiltration capacity for about a year [4]. In a review of 33 patients on this technique, 23 (69%) had return of peritoneal function to previous levels [5].

Use of icodextrin [6], angiotensin-converting enzyme inhibitor or receptor blocker [7], and neutral pH low GDP fluids may have an advantage in prevention of increase in transport characteristics [8, 9] and may help UFF.

Table 6.2 Treatment of ultrafiltration failure (UFF) related to PD peritonitis

Transient UFF during acute stage of PD peritonitis
• Salt and water restriction
• Use of hypertonic solutions like 4.25%
• Use of Icodextrin for long dwell
• Decrease dwell time / increase number of exchanges
• Use of cycler PD
Type 1 UFF associated with recurrent peritonitis
Prevention
• Use of icodextrin
• Use of angiotensin converting enzyme inhibitor/angiotensin receptor blocker
• Use of low GDP neutral pH solutions
Treatment
• Use of icodextrin
• Peritoneal resting

6.6 Important Points

- Peritonitis, especially repeated episodes of peritonitis, may result in ultrafiltration failure.
- Transient ultrafiltration failure may occur as a result of inflammation associated with peritonitis.
- Recurrent peritonitis is likely to result in ultrafiltration failure.
- Type 1 ultrafiltration failure management is challenging and is associated with risk of technique failure.

References

1. ISPD Peritonitis Recommendations. Update on Prevention and Treatment. In: Li PK-T, Szeto CC, Piraino B, de Arteaga J, Fan S, Figueiredo AE, Fish DN, Goffin E, Kim Y-L, Salzer W, Struijk DG, Teitelbaum I, Johnson DW, editors. Peritoneal Dialysis International, vol. 36; 2016. p. 481–508.
2. Devuyst O, Margetts PJ, Topley N. The pathophysiology of the peritoneal membrane. JASN. 2010;21:1077–85.
3. Chow KM, Szeto CC, Kwan BC, Pang WF, Ma T, Leung CB, et al. Randomized controlled study of icodextrin on the treatment of peritoneal dialysis patients during acute peritonitis. Nephrol Dial Transplant. 2014;29:1438–43.
4. de Alvaro F, Castro MJ, Dapena F, Bajo MA, Fernandez-Reyes MJ, Romero JR, Jimenez C, Miranda B, Selgas R. Peritoneal resting is beneficial in peritoneal hyperpermeability and ultrafiltration failure. Adv Perit Dial. 1993;9:56–61.
5. Selgas R, Bajo MA, Castro MJ, et al. Managing ultrafiltration failure by peritoneal resting. Perit Dial Int. 2000;20:595.
6. Davies SJ, Brown EA, Frandsen NE, Rodrigues AS, Rodriguez-Carmona A, Vychytil A, Macnamara E, Ekstrand A, Tranaeus A, Filho JC. EAPOS group: longitudinal membrane function in functionally anuric patients treated with APD: data from EAPOS on the effects of glucose and icodextrin prescription. Kidney Int. 2005;67:1609–15.
7. Kolesnyk I, Noordzij M, Dekker FW, Boeschoten EW, Krediet RT. A positive effect of AII inhibitors on peritoneal membrane function in long-term PD patients. Nephrol Dial Transplant. 2009;24:272–7.
8. Williams JD, Topley N, Craig KJ, Mackenzie RK, Pischetsrieder M, Lage C, Passlick-Deetjen J. Euro balance trial group: the euro-balance trial: the effect of a new biocompatible peritoneal dialysis fluid (balance) on the peritoneal membrane. Kidney Int. 2004;66:408–18.
9. Johnson DW, Brown FG, Clarke M, Boudville N, Elias TJ, Foo MW, Jones B, Kulkarni H, Langham R, Ranganathan D, Schollum J, Suranyi MG, Tan SH, Voss D. balANZ trial investigators: the effect of low glucose degradation product, neutral pH versus standard peritoneal dialysis solutions on peritoneal membrane function: the balANZ trial. Nephrol Dial Transplant. 2012;27:4445–53.

Peritoneal Dialysis-Related Peritonitis and Transfer to Hemodialysis: Challenges

7

B. Karthikeyan, Narayan Prasad, and Krishna Swamy Sampath Kumar

A 48-year-old male, with diabetic kidney disease, hypertension, and end-stage kidney disease (ESKD) who had multiple arteriovenous (AVF) access failures, had been initiated on continuous ambulatory peritoneal dialysis (CAPD) after Tenckhoff catheter insertion by surgical technique. He had good ultrafiltration of 1100 ml/day with three exchanges of 2 L, 2.5% dextrose containing fluid. After 2 years on CAPD, he presented with cloudy effluent and mild abdominal pain for 3 days. His CAPD effluent counts revealed 350 cells/cm^3 of WBC and had polymorphonuclear leucocytes 80%. He was started on intraperitoneal (IP) antibiotics ceftazidime and vancomycin. CAPD fluid culture revealed *Staphylococcus aureus*. Ceftazidime was stopped, and vancomycin was continued. His CAPD effluent had cleared with IP antibiotics, and cell count normalized to 10 cells/cm^3 on day 4 of starting antibiotics.

A month later, he once again presented with cloudy effluent, fever, and abdominal pain. He was started on IP antibiotics, after PD fluid cultures were sent. He had persistent cloudy effluent despite 5 days of IP antibiotics. PD effluent fungal culture revealed *Aspergillus fumigatus*. He was started on IV amphotericin, and the PD catheter was removed. He was temporarily switched to hemodialysis through the right internal jugular vein catheter. He was started on thrice weekly hemodialysis. In the meantime, his abdominal symptoms and fever improved with IV antifungal

B. Karthikeyan
Dr. Rela Institute and Medical Centre, Chennai, Tamil Nadu, India

N. Prasad (✉)
Department of Nephrology, Sanjay Gandhi Postgraduate Institute of Medical Sciences, Lucknow, India

K. S. S. Kumar
Meenakshmi Hospital, Madurai, Tamil Nadu, India

G. Abraham et al. (eds.), *Diagnosis and Management of Complications of Peritoneal Dialysis related Peritonitis*,
https://doi.org/10.1007/978-981-99-2275-8_7

therapy. After 6 weeks, he was assessed for reimplantation of the PD catheter. A computed tomography scan of the abdomen was performed to rule out any intraabdominal collections. After the assessment, the PD catheter was inserted through the laparoscopic technique, which showed no adhesions. After a break-in period of 2 weeks, PD exchanges were done initially with low volume exchanges and then increased to 2 L volume exchanges. He had good ultrafiltration (1.2 L per day) with 3 exchanges of 2.5% dextrose containing fluid each for 4 h dwell and one 7.5% icodextrin night dwell. This is an instance of an ideal case where PD was successfully resumed after catheter removal following refractory fungal peritonitis and temporary switch to hemodialysis.

7.1 Introduction

CAPD is one of the standard therapeutic modalities of renal replacement therapy (RRT) for patients with end-stage kidney disease (ESKD). It is used by almost 15% of the ESKD population worldwide. In some parts of the world, like Hong Kong, PD is the primary modality of choice and is used by 80% of the ESKD population [1]. The main complications of PD are infective and mechanical. The infective complication especially peritonitis is a common cause of technique failure in CAPD patients [2, 3]. This can lead to PD catheter removal and discontinuation of CAPD. These patients may require switching to temporary hemodialysis till the PD catheter is reimplanted. Peritonitis accounts for 30% of treatment failures in PD patients [4]. The timing of removal of the PD catheter depends on the etiology of the peritonitis and its response to treatment.

7.2 PD-Related Peritonitis

PD-related peritonitis is one of the serious complications of PD. Preventing and treating PD-related peritonitis is important in reducing morbidity and mortality. PD-related peritonitis is diagnosed when at least two out of the following three criteria are present [5]:

Cloudy effluent, abdominal pain
Effluent total leucocyte count >100/μL after a dwell time of at least 2 h with >50% of polymorphonuclear leucocytes
Isolation of microorganisms on culture/gram stain

7.3 Peritonitis Rate

Peritonitis rate is usually reported as a number of episodes per patient-year treatment. It can also be expressed as the percentage of patients free of peritonitis in a particular period. The recent ISPD guidelines on peritonitis recommend that the peritonitis rate should not be more than 0.4 episodes per year at risk. And also, the percentage of patients free of peritonitis per unit time should be targeted to more than 80% per year [5].

Table 7.1 Indications of catheter removal and temporary hemodialysis in PD patients

1. Refractory peritonitis
2. Relapsing peritonitis
3. Fungal peritonitis
4. Tunnel or exit site infections with peritonitis

7.4 Peritonitis-Associated Catheter Removal

It is defined as the removal of a PD catheter as part of the treatment of an active peritonitis episode. Patients requiring catheter removal due to peritonitis usually require temporary or permanent switch to hemodialysis as an alternate form of renal replacement therapy.

Peritonitis-Associated Hemodialysis (HD) Transfer
It is defined as the transfer from CAPD to hemodialysis (HD) at any period as a part of the treatment of a peritonitis episode. The various indications for PD catheter removal and peritonitis-associated HD transfer are mentioned in Table 7.1.

Tunnel or Exit Site Infections with Peritonitis
Patients with exit site infections that progress to or occur simultaneously with peritonitis will require catheter removal. For patients who have undergone PD catheter removal for simultaneous exit site or tunnel infection with peritonitis, reimplantation of PD catheter has to be delayed for at least 2–4 weeks [5]. Till then, temporary hemodialysis needs to be instituted for these patients.

7.5 Refractory Peritonitis

Refractory peritonitis is defined as persistent cloudy effluent or PD fluid count of more than 100 cells/cm^3 despite 5 days of appropriate antibiotic therapy. ISPD guidelines recommend that a PD catheter should be removed in cases of refractory peritonitis episode [5].

It is appropriate to wait for the antibiotic effect if the effluent WBC decreases trend toward normal rather than removing the PD catheter. Catheter removal is required early in cases of refractory peritonitis if the patient's condition is deteriorating in order to preserve the peritoneum for future PD and prevent mortality. Attempting to treat refractory peritonitis with prolonged antibiotic therapy without improvement can lead to peritoneal membrane damage. It can also increase the risk of fungal peritonitis and mortality. Hence in cases of refractory peritonitis, PD catheter removal and peritonitis-associated hemodialysis transfer (HD) may be required. Till PD catheter reimplantation, patients need to remain to be on temporary hemodialysis. In some patients, PD catheters cannot be re-implanted due to the after effect of refractory peritonitis and peritoneal membrane failure, and these patients may require permanent transfer to hemodialysis using a vascular access such as tunneled hemodialysis catheter, arteriovenous fistula, or arteriovenous graft.

7.6 Fungal Peritonitis

Fungal peritonitis (FP) is one of the serious complications of PD-associated peritonitis. Peritonitis caused by fungi is associated with higher morbidity and mortality than bacterial peritonitis. Prompt, empirical treatment should be started based on gram stain itself, as identification of fungi can be difficult and take time. Appropriate antifungal therapy based on the sensitivity pattern should be instituted once the correct pathogen is identified. The common pathogens are usually *Candida albicans* and *Candida* non-albicans like *Candida parapsilosis* [6]. The evidence suggests the non-albicans *Candida* species outnumber the *Candida albicans* and other fungal organisms like *Aspergillus fumigatus*, *Aspergillus niger*, etc. Dematiaceous fungi have been reported as causing fungal peritonitis [7, 8]. Other fungi like mucormycosis and aspergillosis also can cause severe refractory peritonitis. Fungal peritonitis is associated with peritoneal membrane damage and subsequent risk of technique failure in PD patients. Hence, catheter removal is recommended in fungal peritonitis as soon as the diagnosis is made. Appropriate antifungal treatment is recommended for at least 2 weeks after catheter removal. The mortality rate without catheter removal approaches between 50% to 91%, so catheter removal remains the cornerstone in managing fungal peritonitis [7–9]. After an episode of FP, no more than 35% of patients are able to continue PD or have the technique re-established, and apart from the patients who die, this is most often because of complications such as peritoneal adhesions, abscess formation, or progressive sclerosing peritonitis. Temporary hemodialysis needs to be instituted till the reinsertion of PD catheter. Attempts at reimplantation of the permanent PD catheter can be made after a waiting period of 4–6 weeks. Most refractory peritonitis episodes are due to fungal peritonitis. In some cases, PD catheter reinsertion could not be done due to the persistent abdominal pain and non-resolving ascites after peritonitis [10]. In these patients, permanent transfer to hemodialysis may be required. Failure to resume the PD occurs in up to 40% of patients with fungal peritonitis.

7.7 Relapsing Peritonitis

Relapsing peritonitis is defined as a peritonitis episode that occurs within 4 weeks of completion of therapy of a prior peritonitis episode with the same organism. Many retrospective studies report that relapsing peritonitis is associated with a lower rate of cure when compared to non-relapsing peritonitis. It is also associated with a higher risk of ultrafiltration and technique failure [11]. ISPD guidelines recommend the timely removal of PD catheters in relapsing peritonitis.

7.8 Recurrent Peritonitis

Recurrent peritonitis is defined as a peritonitis episode that occurs within 4 weeks of completion of therapy of a prior peritonitis episode but with a different organism. This has a worse prognosis than relapsing peritonitis, and timely catheter removal is indicated in this peritonitis [12].

7.9 Repeat Peritonitis

Repeat peritonitis is defined as a peritonitis episode that occurs with the same organism more than 4 weeks after the completion of therapy of the previous episode. Simultaneous removal and reinsertion of PD catheter can be done in cases of relapsing, recurrent, and repeat peritonitis after the PD effluent culture is negative with a cell count less than 100 cells/cm^3. There should not be associated exit or tunnel infection during this procedure [13]. Simultaneous removal and re-implantation should be carried out only if culture reports are negative and cell count of the effluent <100 cells/cm^3 have to be done under antibiotic coverage. It is not appropriate to attempt simultaneous removal and reimplantation of the catheter if the bacterial culture is still positive. If the culture is positive or if there is associated exit site or tunnel infection, simultaneous catheter removal and reinsertion should not be attempted. These patients require PD catheter removal and temporary transfer to hemodialysis.

Catheter removal may be considered for repeat peritonitis, mycobacterial peritonitis, and peritonitis with multiple enteric organisms. After PD catheter removal, a patient needs to be instituted on temporary hemodialysis till the PD catheter is reinserted and PD is resumed.

7.10 Temporary HD after PD Catheter Removal

After removal of the PD catheter due to peritonitis, the patient needs to be started on the alternate form of renal replacement therapy, i.e., hemodialysis. Access for initiating hemodialysis may be either temporary or permanent HD catheter, and in a few of the patients, previously created arteriovenous fistula can be used for initiating hemodialysis. Patients who were started on hemodialysis through permanent access reported better survival than those who began on HD through temporary access [14].

7.11 Outcomes of Patients after Transferring to HD

Although the transition from PD to HD is common after a peritonitis episode, the outcomes are a little known. There is increased mortality after the immediate transition to HD, probably related to the recent peritonitis episode. Patients with refractory peritonitis may have persistent abdominal symptoms or non-resolving ascites, preventing them from resuming CAPD [10]. The mortality in the first year of refractory peritonitis is very high (Table 7.2).

In a study by Nadeau-Fredette et al. [15], where they analyzed the multinational registry data to assess the risk factors and mortality rate after transfer to HD from PD, they found mortality risk was increased in these patients within the first 30 days of transfer to HD. The risk factors for increased mortality after HD transfer are older age, patients on PD for more than 3 years, female sex compared to the male sex, and patients with diabetic nephropathy and peritonitis as a cause of HD transfer. The data from Australian and New Zealand Dialysis and Transplant (ANZDATA) registry found that those transferring to HD for

Table 7.2 Common causes of PD technique failure and risk factors for mortality during transfer to HD

Common cause of technique failure	Risk factors of mortality during HD transfer
PD peritonitis Mechanical problems Inadequate dialysis (can follow an episode of peritonitis)	Older age Long PD vintage period Female sex Infection as a cause of technique failure Diabetic nephropathy

peritonitis had a higher risk of early mortality than those who transfer to HD for other reasons like inadequate dialysis or mechanical reasons. In a study by Thammishetti et al. [10], almost 48% of patients who got transferred to hemodialysis after an episode of refractory peritonitis died within the first year of catheter removal or CAPD discontinuation. Nearly 33% of patients died within 3 months of transfer to HD. It is still not known clearly why there is high mortality during the first year after HD transfer. It may be due to multiple causes like cardiovascular events, HD catheter-related bacteremia, sepsis, frequent hospitalizations, or non-resolving peritonitis.

7.12 Re-initiation of PD after Temporary HD

Notwithstanding the fact that peritonitis can damage the peritoneal membrane, there are scientific evidences about the feasibility of resuming successful PD after an episode of peritonitis. ISPD guidelines recommend that the PD catheter reimplantation can be attempted after at least 2 to 4 weeks of rest following peritonitis (Fig. 7.1). The best evidence to date regarding successful re-initiation of PD after temporary HD is provided by Cho et al. [16]. This group analyzed the data from the ANZDATA registry and found that only 16.7% of peritonitis episodes warranted catheter removal and transfer to HD. Of these, only 18.3% returned to PD, and the rest continued permanently on HD. The group of patients who restarted on PD had outcomes similar to those who remained on PD without peritonitis and those who transferred permanently to HD.

Considering all these factors, PD can be successfully restarted in a small but significant cohort of patients who undergo catheter removal and require hemodialysis following peritonitis [17–22]. Re-implantation of PD after temporary HD in these patients can be followed by ultrafiltration failure (UFF), need for additional exchanges, or another episode of refractory peritonitis. In patients who permanently transfer to HD, the best outcomes are achieved in those who use permanent vascular access [14].

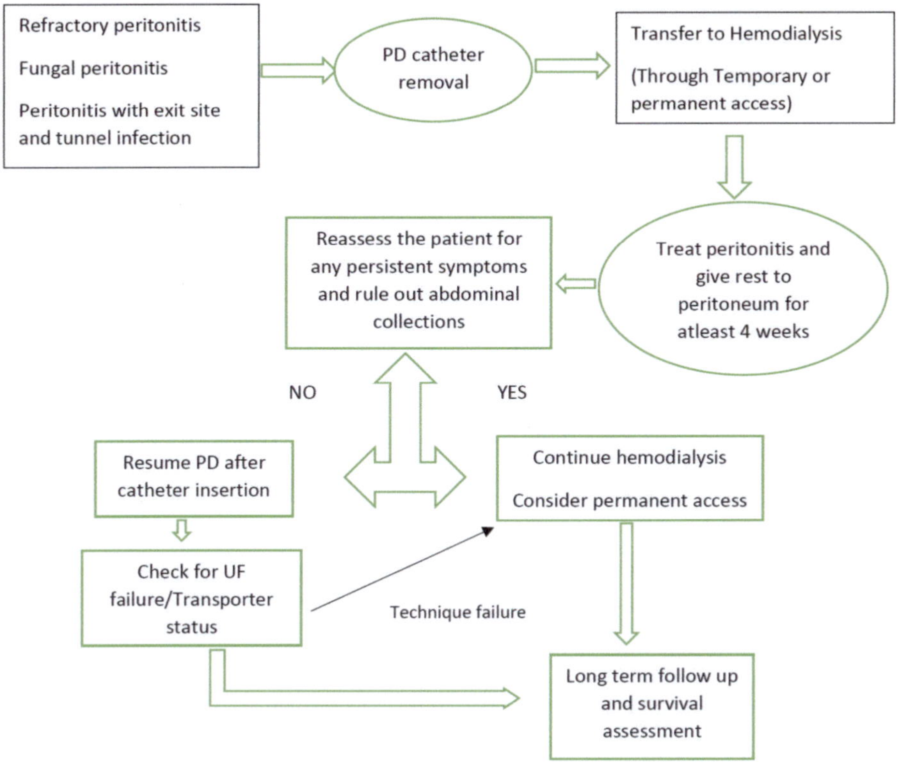

Fig. 7.1 Flow chart depicting indications, outcomes, and follow-up in peritonitis-associated HD transfer

7.13 Important Points

- Peritonitis-associated transfer of patients to HD is required in cases of refractory peritonitis, fungal peritonitis, and peritonitis associated with simultaneous exit or tunnel infections.
- In cases of relapsing, recurrent, and repeat peritonitis, after the culture is negative, simultaneous catheter removal and reinsertion can be done.
- Simultaneous removal and reinsertion are not advisable if the culture is positive, and in these groups of patients, catheter removal and transfer to HD may be necessary.
- Patients with polymicrobial peritonitis and mycobacterial peritonitis may require PD catheter removal and transfer to HD.

- Peritonitis-associated transfer to HD is associated with an increased risk of technique failure and mortality.
- Although a small cohort of patients can resume PD after a rest of at least 4 weeks, ultrafiltration failure and change in transporter status may occur.
- Early catheter removal and aggressive treatment of peritonitis help preserve the peritoneum to restart PD and have better outcome.

References

1. Jain AK, Blake P, Cordy P, Garg AX. Global trends in rates of peritoneal dialysis. J Am Soc Nephrol JASN. 2012 Mar;23(3):533–44.
2. Shen JI, Mitani AA, Saxena AB, Goldstein BA, Winkelmayer WC. Determinants of peritoneal dialysis technique failure in incident US patients. Perit Dial Int J Int Soc Perit Dial. 2013;33(2):155–66.
3. Hsieh YP, Chang CC, Wang SC, Wen YK, Chiu PF, Yang Y. Predictors for and impact of high peritonitis rate in Taiwanese continuous ambulatory peritoneal dialysis patients. Int Urol Nephrol. 2015 Jan;47(1):183–9.
4. Liu X, Qin A, Zhou H, He X, Cader S, Wang S, et al. Novel predictors and risk score of treatment failure in peritoneal dialysis-related peritonitis. Front Med. 2021 Mar;19(8):639744.
5. Li PKT, Chow KM, Cho Y, Fan S, Figueiredo AE, Harris T, et al. ISPD peritonitis guideline recommendations: 2022 update on prevention and treatment. Perit Dial Int J Int Soc Perit Dial. 2022 Mar;42(2):110–53.
6. Auricchio S, Giovenzana ME, Pozzi M, Galassi A, Santorelli G, Dozio B, et al. Fungal peritonitis in peritoneal dialysis: a 34-year single Centre evaluation. Clin Kidney J. 2018 Dec;11(6):874–80.
7. Prasad KN, Prasad N, Gupta A, Sharma RK, Verma AK, Ayyagari A. Fungal peritonitis in patients on continuous ambulatory peritoneal dialysis: a single Centre Indian experience. J Infect. 2004 Jan;48(1):96–101.
8. Wang AY, Yu AW, Li PK, Lam PK, Leung CB, Lai KN, et al. Factors predicting outcome of fungal peritonitis in peritoneal dialysis: analysis of a 9-year experience of fungal peritonitis in a single center. Am J Kidney Dis Off J Natl Kidney Found. 2000 Dec;36(6):1183–92.
9. Prasad N, Gupta A. Fungal peritonitis in peritoneal dialysis patients. Perit Dial Int. 2005 May-Jun;25(3):207–22.
10. Thammishetti V, Kaul A, Bhadauria DS, Balasubramanian K, Prasad N, Gupta A, et al. A retrospective analysis of etiology and outcomes of refractory CAPD peritonitis in a tertiary care center from North India. Perit Dial Int J Int Soc Perit Dial. 2018 Dec;38(6):441–6.
11. Szeto CC, Kwan BCH, Chow KM, Law MC, Pang WF, Chung KY, et al. Recurrent and relapsing peritonitis: causative organisms and response to treatment. Am J Kidney Dis Off J Natl Kidney Found. 2009 Oct;54(4):702–10.
12. Burke M, Hawley CM, Badve SV, McDonald SP, Brown FG, Boudville N, et al. Relapsing and recurrent peritoneal dialysis-associated peritonitis: a multicenter registry study. Am J Kidney Dis Off J Natl Kidney Found. 2011 Sep;58(3):429–36.
13. Crabtree JH, Shrestha BM, Chow KM, Figueiredo AE, Povlsen JV, Wilkie M, et al. Creating and maintaining optimal peritoneal dialysis access in the adult patient: 2019 update. Perit Dial Int J Int Soc Perit Dial. 2019 Oct;39(5):414–36.
14. Pajek J, Hutchison AJ, Bhutani S, Brenchley PEC, Hurst H, Perme MP, et al. Outcomes of peritoneal dialysis patients and switching to haemodialysis: a competing risks analysis. Perit Dial Int J Int Soc Perit Dial. 2014 May;34(3):289–98.

15. Nadeau-Fredette AC, Sukul N, Lambie M, Perl J, Davies S, Johnson DW, et al. Mortality trends after transfer from peritoneal dialysis to Haemodialysis. Kidney Int Rep. 2022 May;7(5):1062–73.
16. Cho Y, Badve SV, Hawley CM, McDonald SP, Brown FG, Boudville N, et al. Peritoneal dialysis outcomes after temporary haemodialysis transfer for peritonitis. Nephrol Dial Transplant. - Eur Ren Assoc. 2014 Oct;29(10):1940–7.
17. Szeto CC, Chow KM, Wong TYH, Leung CB, Wang AYM, Lui SF, et al. Feasibility of resuming peritoneal dialysis after severe peritonitis and Tenckhoff catheter removal. J Am Soc Nephrol JASN. 2002 Apr;13(4):1040–5.
18. Choi P, Nemati E, Banerjee A, Preston E, Levy J, Brown E. Peritoneal dialysis catheter removal for acute peritonitis: a retrospective analysis of factors associated with catheter removal and prolonged postoperative hospitalization. Am J Kidney Dis. 2004 Jan;43(1):103–11.
19. Ram R, Swarnalatha G, Dakshinamurty KV. Re-initiation of peritoneal dialysis after catheter removal for refractory peritonitis. J Nephrol. 2014 Aug;27(4):445–9.
20. Chediak Terán C, Sosa Barrios RH, Burguera Vion V, Fernández Lucas M, Rivera Gorrín ME. Resuming peritoneal dialysis after catheter removal due to complicated peritonitis. Clin Exp Nephrol. 2020 Apr;24(4):349–55.
21. Troidle L, Gorban-Brennan N, Finkelstein FO. Outcome of patients on chronic peritoneal dialysis undergoing peritoneal catheter removal because of peritonitis. Adv Perit Dial Conf Perit Dial. 2005;21:98–101.
22. Donovan K, Carrington C. Peritoneal dialysis outcomes after temporary haemodialysis for peritonitis–influence on current practice. Nephrol Dial Transplant 2014 Oct;29(10):1803–5.

Relapsing and Refractory Peritonitis Special Challenge

8

Sreelatha, Maithrayie Kumaresan, and Anil Bhalla

8.1 PD Peritonitis in an Immunocompromised Patient

A 37-year-old hypertensive male was initiated on CAPD as renal replacement therapy (RRT) for chronic kidney disease (CKD) G5, secondary to chronic glomerulonephritis. He underwent diseased donor renal transplantation elsewhere, which rejected in less than a year, and hence he subsequently returned to CAPD using double bag disposable system. He was admitted with signs and symptoms of peritonitis, diarrhea, and poor appetite for 2 weeks. There was no tunnel infection and exit site was healthy. He had two episodes of peritonitis due to *Pseudomonas aeruginosa* which responded to intraperitoneal ceftriaxone. On admission, investigations showed hemoglobin 6 gm/dI, WBC count 9600 cell/mm^3, urea 119 mg/dI, creatinine 15.2 mg/dI, sodium 135 mmol/l, potassium 4.3 mmol/l, bicarbonate 27 mmol/It, chloride 105 mmol/It, calcium 10.3 mg/dl, iPTH 1305 pg/ml and vitamin 25 (OH) D3 19 ng/ml, total serum protein 7.6gm/dI, albumin 3.6gm/dI, and ESR 150 mm/h. His serology was negative for HbsAg, anti-HCV antibody, and HIV. The dialysis effluent cell count was 480cells/mm^3 with predominantly polymorphonuclear leukocytosis. The peritonitis was due to non-fermenting gram-negative bacilli. He was treated initially with intraperitoneal (IP) cefazolin, ceftazidime, and ciprofloxacin as per sensitivity report. However, his peritonitis did not respond to

Sreelatha (✉)
Kozhikode Medical College and Hospital, Kozhikode, India

M. Kumaresan
Gangaram Hospital New Delhi, New Delhi, India

A. Bhalla
University Hospital Lewisham, London, UK

G. Abraham et al. (eds.), *Diagnosis and Management of Complications of Peritoneal Dialysis related Peritonitis*,
https://doi.org/10.1007/978-981-99-2275-8_8

different combination of IP antibiotics, and he remained toxic with severe abdominal pain and required PD catheter removal. He was switched to hemodialysis through dual lumen right-sided jugular catheter, and an arteriovenous fistula (AVF) was created. As he had persistent spikes of fever despite treatment with appropriate antibiotics, CT-guided drainage of a collection in pelvis and subhepatic region was undertaken, which on culture did not grow any organisms. He continued to have high spiking fever despite drainage of ascites was done and empiric antitubercular therapy with PO isoniazid 150 mg once daily, PO rifampicin 600 mg once daily, and pyrazinamide 1gm once daily and PO levofloxacin 500 mg once daily was initiated along with vitamin B6. With this regimen, he became afebrile over the next 2 weeks. Patient wanted to continue RRT with CAPD. Hence, he underwent laparoscopy to attempt reimplantation of a swan neck Tenckhoff catheter [1]. However, this showed presence of extensive intraperitoneal adhesions and septations and the attempt was aborted (Fig. 8.1).

Andrews et al. have shown patients on CAPD who are immunosuppressed with previous kidney transplantation, glomerulonephritis, systemic lupus erythematosus, and other vasculitis had increased likelihood of PD peritonitis [2]. These patients required more hospitalization and several days off CAPD, and there was increased requirement of laparotomy surgeries to remove infected catheters. Immunosuppression was also associated with high infection rate due to *Staphylococcus aureus* and fungi contributing to increase morbidity. Our patient had culture negative episodes of refractory peritonitis and required catheter removal along with antituberculous drug therapy for resolution unmasking an undiagnosed mycobacterium tuberculosis. Besides the immunosuppressant effect of CKD, additional immunosuppressive medications may further impair both cellular and humoral immunity.

A patient who is immunosuppressed has high risk of recurrent peritonitis and refractive peritonitis requiring PD catheter removal to prevent morbidity and

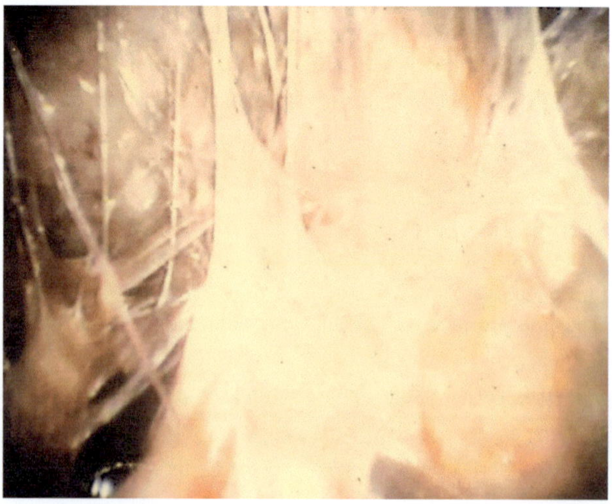

Fig. 8.1 Laparoscopic examination showing extensive peritoneal adhesions

mortality. Severe recurrent peritonitis leads to formation of extensive adhesions, and reimplantation of the catheter will be fraught with many difficulties as discussed in the above patient. Current immunosuppression or a recent history of immunosuppression appeared to be equally potent risk factors for infection. However, being on immunosuppressive therapy per se is not a contraindication for CAPD initiation.

Immunosuppressed individuals are at an increased risk of developing episodes of peritonitis and also refractory peritonitis. Besides the immunosuppressant effects of renal failure, immunosuppressive therapy may further impair the immunity of the patient. Steroids even at low doses may contribute to inadequate response to antibiotics and may necessitate removal of the catheter for resolution of peritonitis. In addition, immunosuppression may further decrease the immune response and increase the severity of peritonitis. So, immunosuppression appears to be one of the important risk factors for refractory peritonitis.

8.2 Peritoneal Adhesions Following Recurrent or Severe Peritonitis

Mr. X 60-year-old gentleman with diabetic kidney disease and CKD G 5 was initiated on RRT with CAPD. He had significant macrovascular complications of diabetes in the form of coronary artery disease and peripheral vascular disease. His blood sugars were always uncontrolled. After 2 months of being on CAPD, he developed abdominal pain with cloudy effluent. His PD fluid total leukocyte count was 6700 cells/ml, with >90% polymorphonuclear leukocytes. Diagnosis of PD peritonitis was made and he was started on treatment with IP vancomycin and ceftazidime, after PD fluid effluent was sent for gram stain and culture with sensitivity. No other etiological factors could be identified, apart from uncontrolled diabetes. After 72 h, the cultures were still sterile. On the fifth day, repeat PD effluent tests showed 50% reduction in total leukocyte count to 3000/ml and polymorphonuclear leukocytes to 20%. As the patient has attained a partial remission with vancomycin and ceftazidime, he was continued on the same IP antibiotics along with oral fluconazole for antifungal prophylaxis. However, his symptoms worsened over the next few days and PD fluid leukocyte count had again increased to 4500/ml. Samples of PD fluid effluent sent for cultures again remained sterile. Fungal cultures and mycobacterial cultures were also negative. The PD catheter was removed and the patient was initiated on hemodialysis. His fever and abdominal pain persisted in spite of catheter removal, and hence, laparoscopic evaluation of peritoneal cavity was done. On laparoscopy, an occult pelvic collection was seen, which was drained and sent for bacterial, fungal, and mycobacterial cultures. There were also extensive adhesions in the peritoneal cavity. The patient was initiated on empirical antitubercular therapy, pending mycobacterial cultures. The patient responded over the next 2 weeks with complete resolution of symptoms. The culture grew atypical mycobacteria [3]. Such protracted peritonitis episodes can lead to formation of peritoneal adhesions, peritoneal inflammation with loss of mesothelial cells, and ultrafiltration failure. Protracted peritonitis with culture negativity or persistence of symptoms after appropriate antibiotic therapy should arouse suspicion of *mycobacterium tuberculosis* or atypical mycobacterial infection, and appropriate treatment should be instituted. Early initiation of anti-mycobacterial therapy will prevent the formation of adhesions, and patient can be reinitiated on CAPD after a few weeks.

Tuberculous peritonitis is often underdiagnosed or diagnosed very late. Symptoms are commonly similar to bacterial peritonitis. Constitutional systemic symptoms are common in all patients due to uremia. PD fluid cell count need not be always lymphocyte predominant. Tuberculin skin test is often negative because of anergy in CKD patients. Diagnosis requires a high index of suspicion. All these are diagnostic challenges in TB peritonitis. There is a paucity of research on IP drug dosing for automated PD (APD) which can interfere with treatment adequacy and incomplete treatment. Randomized controlled trials are needed to compare the efficacy and safety of different antibiotic regimens in APD. In cases of protracted peritonitis with cultures being negative or persistence of symptoms after appropriate antibiotic therapy, there should be clinical suspicion of mycobacterium tuberculosis, and appropriate therapy should be instituted.

Fungal peritonitis is a serious complication of chronic peritoneal dialysis, associated with high morbidity and mortality. It is associated with peritoneal adhesions, sclerosis, and irreversible membrane damage leading to significant risk of technique failure. Up to 40% patients are unable to resume PD requiring transfer to hemodialysis. The mortality rate varies from15% to 50%. Several centers are still not using antifungal prophylaxis during antibiotic treatment for bacterial peritonitis. This leads to increased risk of fungal peritonitis. Multiple episodes of bacterial peritonitis predispose to fungal infection. In view of the high biofilm production observed in fungal peritonitis, immediate catheter removal is recommended as the best option to reduce the high mortality of fungal peritonitis, and patient should be initiated on appropriate antifungal therapy. Patient also requires prolonged treatment with antifungal drugs, at least 2 weeks after removal of PD catheter. So, fungal peritonitis is a real challenge for a PD program.

8.3 Multiple Episodes of Peritonitis

Multiple episodes of peritonitis can lead to deleterious functional alterations in the peritoneal membrane with loss of dialysis capacity leading to increase in morbidity and mortality.

A 51-year-old married woman, with type 2 diabetes mellitus for 4 years, hypothyroidism, past paralytic poliomyelitis of the right leg, chronic kidney disease (CKD) due to autosomal dominant polycystic kidney disease, and a clipped cerebral aneurysm was referred to us following 21 episodes of peritonitis in a span of 76 months while on CAPD. She was switched to continuous ambulatory PD (CAPD) due to multiple access failures on hemodialysis (HD). The patient and her supportive spouse were trained to do the procedure of CAPD 4 times a day. She had 11 episodes of culture-negative peritonitis and 10 episodes of culture-positive peritonitis with *Enterococcus faecalis*, *Staphylococcus saprophyticus*, and *Escherichia coli*.

These episodes were several episodes of recurrent peritonitis, one episode of relapsing peritonitis, and one episode of refractory peritonitis, in keeping with the definition as per International Society of Peritoneal Dialysis.

She had no previous exit site or tunnel infection. She developed an episode of refractory peritonitis; hence CAPD was discontinued and switched to HD using a temporary jugular access. On examination, her supine blood pressure was 80/50 mmHg, she had no abdominal tenderness, the catheter exit site was not infected, and there was no tunnel tenderness. A clear dialysate effluent fluid that drained after 4 h of indwell time was sent for culture, and it showed no growth after 48 h. It was also negative by polymerase chain reaction (Gene XPert PCR) for *Mycobacterium tuberculosis*. Ultrasound of the tunnel did not show any collection. We proceeded with a laparoscopic examination of the peritoneal cavity which showed a normal-appearing peritoneum, a cirrhotic liver, and minimal ascites without adhesions. Catheter-tip biofilm culture isolated *Enterococcus casseliflavus*. Two weeks later, CAPD was reinitiated and she received 2 g of intraperitoneal immunoglobulin in two separate doses with a dwell of 6 h as treatment for recurrent peritonitis in the form of empirical therapy. She is currently on APD. The laparoscopic evaluation of the peritoneum helped to assess the presence of adhesions after peritonitis episodes in this patient with 21 episodes of peritonitis, and the biofilm culture of the catheter tip was helpful in identifying the organism in otherwise culture negative peritonitis.

In PD patients, there is activation of peritoneal macrophages and loss of mesothelial cells, macrophages, and immunoglobulins, thereby leading to impaired host defense and hence increase susceptibility to infection. Uremia, peritonitis, volume loading, the presence of a catheter, and the PD fluid all initiate recruitment and activation of peritoneal cells such as macrophages, mast cells, mesothelial cells, fibroblasts, and endothelial cells. This leads to the development of angiogenesis, fibrosis, and membrane failure.

The ISPD recommends that timely catheter removal be considered for relapsing, recurrent, or refractory peritonitis episodes. Furthermore, it is recommended that the PD catheter be removed promptly in refractory peritonitis episodes to avoid membrane failure and especially mortality. Recurrent PD peritonitis due to biofilm formation on the catheter requires prompt removal of the catheter for resolution of the infection.

4. We report a rare and unusual case that occurred in 1993 in which a young male patient with Epstein's syndrome and severe thrombocytopenia had two episodes of peritonitis with intraperitoneal hemorrhage whose management was very complex. There was co-infection with *Candida albicans*. The patient later required two laparotomy surgeries for removal of catheter and drainage of ascites infected with *Mycobacterium tuberculosis*. Faced with the challenging situation, in desperation before removal of the catheter intraperitoneal fluconazole and netilmicin along with oral flucytosine was tried but proved to be futile. Addition of IP amphotericin in an effort to save the catheter was unsuccessful. All this increased the duration of hospitalization, morbidity, malnutrition, and stress of abdominal surgery. This case was discussed at the dialysis meeting at Denver, Colorado, 1997 as a complex clinicopathologic conference (CPC) case [4].

8.4 Important Points

1. Co-infection peritonitis with protracted course leading to peritoneal adhesions and abscesses produce irreversible peritoneal damage.
2. Peritonitis in CAPD patients with immunosuppressive therapy is difficult to treat and is faced with challenges.
3. For bio-film formation of the catheters, the best management option is replacement of catheter after cure of peritonitis.
4. Prior antibiotic therapy is a risk factor for fungal peritonitis.

References

1. Ignatius A, Kalra D, Prasad N, Gupta A. Refractory Peritonitis in a CAPD Patient on Immunosuppression. Ind J Perit Dial. 2006;11:37–9.
2. Andrews PA, Warr KJ, Hicks JA, Cameron JS. Impaired outcome of continuous ambulatory peritoneal dialysis in immunocompromised patients. Nephrol Dial Transplantation. 1996;11:1104–8.
3. Nagarajan P, et al. Adhesions following recurrent peritonitis in a failed allograft recipient. Ind J Perit Dial, [Sl]. 2006:35–6. Available at: http://52.172.159.94/index.php/ijpd/article/view/51250
4. Twardowski ZJ, Zimmerman S, Abraham G. Was CAPD the answer to this patient's complex problems? Perit Dial Int. 1997;17:630–536.

Reimplantation and Reinitiation of Peritoneal Dialysis after Catheter Removal for Refractory Peritonitis

9

Ram R, Gomathy Sankara Narayana Iyer, Sudha Teresa, and Priyanka Govindhan

A 45 years old gentleman was diagnosed to have chronic glomerulonephritis with and end-stage kidney disease (ESKD). He was initiated on peritoneal dialysis in March 2014 and on three exchanges of 1.5% dextrose solution. The ultrafiltrate was 1.2 liter per day, and the residual urine output was 750 mL/d and assumed a high average transporter status. The peritoneal equilibration test (PET) showed him to be a high average transporter. In November 2014, he developed a refractory peritonitis which grown *Pseudomonas aeruginosa*, following which the peritoneal dialysis catheter was removed and he was shifted to hemodialysis. He suffered refractory peritonitis and exit site infection due to *Pseudomonas aeruginosa*, and the peritoneal dialysis catheter had to be removed. Subsequently, evaluation including peritoneography and computerized scan (CT) did not show any adhesions in the peritoneum. Patient had to be transferred to hemodialysis. After peritoneal scintigraphy and computerized tomography, scan of abdomen showed no adhesions. Hence, in January 2015, the peritoneal dialysis catheter was reinserted. He was continued on three exchanges of 1.5% dextrose solution. The ultrafiltrate was 800 mL/d and the residual urine output was 600 mL/d. The repeat peritoneal equilibration test showed again high average transporter status. 2 years later in February

R. R (✉)
Sri Venkateswara Institute of Medical Sciences, Tirupati, India

G. S. N. Iyer
TD Medical College Allepy, Alappuzha, India

S. Teresa
MGM Hospital, Chennai, Tamil Nadu, India

P. Govindhan
Nephrologic Clinic Fort Collims, University of Colorado, Boulder, CO, USA

G. Abraham et al. (eds.), *Diagnosis and Management of Complications of Peritoneal Dialysis related Peritonitis*,
https://doi.org/10.1007/978-981-99-2275-8_9

2017, patient suffered another episode of refractory peritonitis, and the peritoneal dialysis catheter had to be removed. After ruling out peritoneal adhesions, the peritoneal dialysis catheter was reintroduced confirming the absence of adhesions on peritoneal scintigraphy and CT scan abdomen. The peritoneal dialysis catheter was again reinserted. Meanwhile, an arteriovenous fistula was also secured. In February 2018, the residual renal function was 100 mL/fd, and the PET revealed that he has a low average transporter.

In India, proportion of patients on peritoneal dialysis in our country is 18–20% [1]. The concept of reinitiation of PD has not gained momentum in our country.

In a patient undergoing peritoneal dialysis (PD), catheter removal during the course of an episode of severe peritonitis is to prevent its two major consequences of uncontrolled peritonitis, namely, death and irreversible injury to the peritoneal membrane, the latter precluding future continuation of PD therapy [2]. The other indications for catheter removal are refractory peritonitis, relapsing peritonitis, refractory exit site and tunnel infection, and fungal peritonitis. Catheter removal may also be considered for repeat peritonitis, mycobacterial peritonitis, and multiple enteric organisms [3].

Catheter removal for peritonitis renders fair to good results when indicated for reasons other than the clinical aggressiveness of the infection, as in uncomplicated relapsing or catheter-dependent peritonitis. These settings allow a chance to induce clinical remission of the infection with antibiotics, permitting removal or even one-step catheter exchange [4] in the absence of peritoneal inflammation. Thus, removal of the catheter may be lifesaving in many patients of severe peritonitis, yet though this step is associated with high mortality rates. Peritonitis with catheter removal is usually associated with significantly higher mortality rates [5–8] than those reported for PD-related peritonitis overall [7, 9–11]. Patients who survive this serious (in terms of both risk and suffering) complication stand in a disadvantageous position both clinically and psychologically find themselves in poor clinical and psychological condition [2]. The available information literature on this reveals that [2] reinitiation of PD does not happen successfully either due to patient preference or due to clinician's inertia for empiric reasons or due to evidence of irreversible peritoneal injury. a high proportion of patients whose catheters were removed were unable to successfully reinitiate PD, due to irreversible peritoneal injury or to decisions by the patient or the nephrologist, the latter for empiric reasons.

A recollection of some of the definitions are as follows:

(IA). Peritonitis: Presence of any two of the following: (a) symptoms and signs of peritoneal inflammation, (b) cloudy peritoneal fluid effluent with an elevated peritoneal fluid leucocyte count (more than 100/μL) due predominantly (more than 50%) to neutrophils, and (c) demonstration of bacteria in the peritoneal fluid by Gram's stain or culture

(II.B) Refractory peritonitis: Failure of the peritoneal effluent fluid to clear after 5 days of appropriate antibiotics [3]

(III. C) Technique failure: Permanent transfer to hemodialysis

Reinitiation of PD

The decision to reinitiate PD should be taken solely by the patient. The nephrology team treating the patient should limit the influence only to inform them the possibility of reinitiation of PD. Only after patients had convinced themselves and expressed willingness for PD, further investigations should be done to proceed with reinsertion of PD catheter once the patient is fully convinced of its pros and cons. In all patients, a minimum of 4 weeks should elapse after catheter removal, before a new one be removed and reinserted. In one study, the reported mean interval after the removal of catheter and attempt of reinsertion was 50.4 days [12]. After 2009, all patients were subjected to peritoneal scintigraphy, and computerized tomography is considered as ideal investigations to detect peritoneal adhesions prior to attempting catheter reinsertion to assess the presence of adhesions in the abdomen.

9.1 Peritoneal Scintigraphy

The peritoneal scintigraphy is performed by mixing 2.0 mCi technetium-99 m sulfur colloid in 2 L 2.5% dextrose peritoneal dialysis solution and then infusing the same using a 14-gauge intravenous cannula under aseptic conditions precautions. Scintigraphic views are obtained using a large field of view scintillation camera set at 140 keV photopeak, with a 20% window, and equipped with a low energy parallel-hole collimator. Starting at the time of infusion, a dynamic series of 1 min/frame images centered on the diaphragmatic region were obtained for15 min. Static anterior, posterior, and lateral views of the abdomen were then obtained at post infusion and post ambulatory phases and after draining out the radiolabeled dialysate. A normal scan should demonstrate free flow of dialysate fluid throughout the peritoneal cavity, outlining the intraperitoneal recesses (Fig. 9.1). A nonuniform distribution of the dialysate fluid, with most of it confining to the central part of the abdomen in several loculations (Fig. 9.2), suggests the presence of adhesions. The loculated tracer accumulation persistent even after draining of dialysate fluid confirms the presence of adhesions [13].

The reinsertion of catheter should be done either by open surgery or by laparoscopy.

The previous studies [6, 8, 12, 14, 15] on reinsertion of peritoneal dialysis are reported in Table 9.1. The previous studies identified severe peritonitis, dialysis vintage, and increasing patient age as factors that predicted the technique failure.

In our program, the organisms which caused refractory peritonitis were fungal: 7 (22.5%); *Pseudomonas aeruginosa*: 4 (12.9%); *Escherichia coli*: 3 (9.6%); *Staphylococcus aureus*; coagulase negative staphylococcus and *Mycobacterium tuberculosis*: 2 (6.4%) each; and *Acinetobacter baumannii* and *Klebsiella pneumonia*: 1 (3.2%) each. It was culture negative in 9 (29%) patients. Also in our program, the decision of reinitiation of PD was mainly taken by the patient not influenced by us. The decision was taken by the patient. Early removal of catheter on day 5 or 6, a mean interval of 50.4 days after the removal of catheter, use of peritoneal scintigraphy to rule out adhesions, and reinsertion of catheter by open surgery might have

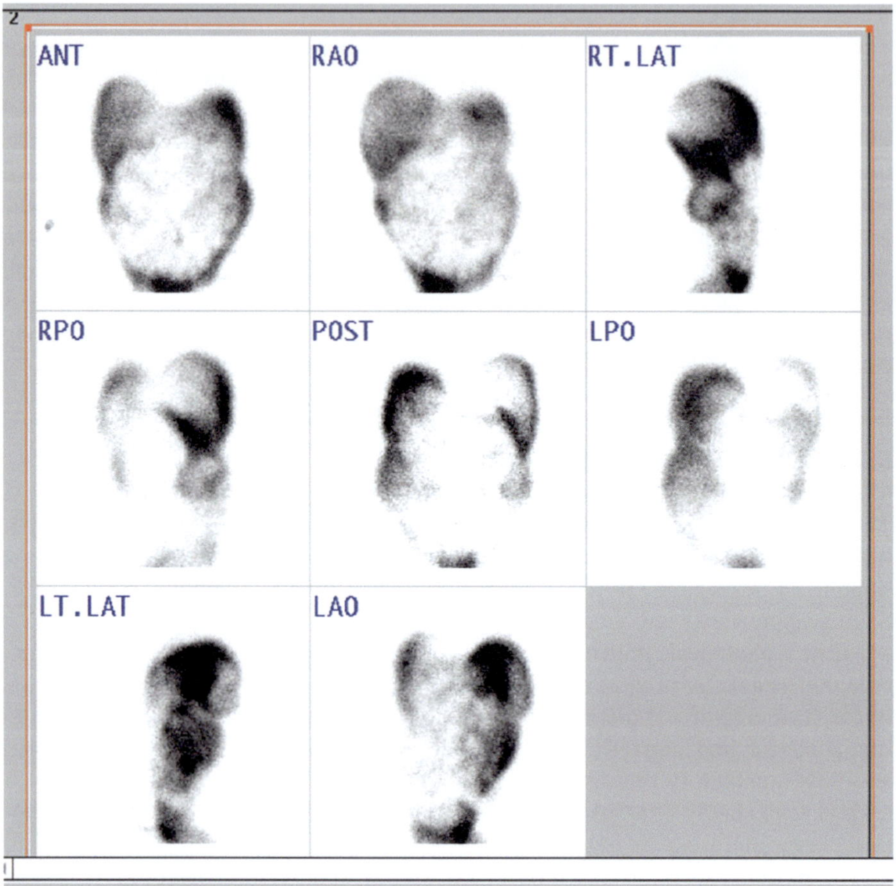

Fig. 9.1 Free flow of dialysate fluid throughout the peritoneal cavity, outlining the intraperitoneal recesses

contributed to successful reinitiation of PD in our patients. We could not find any difference in the effect of organism causing peritonitis on reinitiation of PD. However, it was opined that the agents with aggressive and/or persistent infections (yeast and surgical enteric peritonitis) might impede reinitiation of PD [2]. A previous study has reported an increase in D/P creatinine ratio after reinitiation of PD [6]. We also observed a similar increase in the proportion of high and high average transporters after reinitiation (47.61%) than before (33.33%). This change from low and low average transporter to high and high average transporter status could be due to long-term peritoneal dialysis resulting in high solute transport status (Type 1

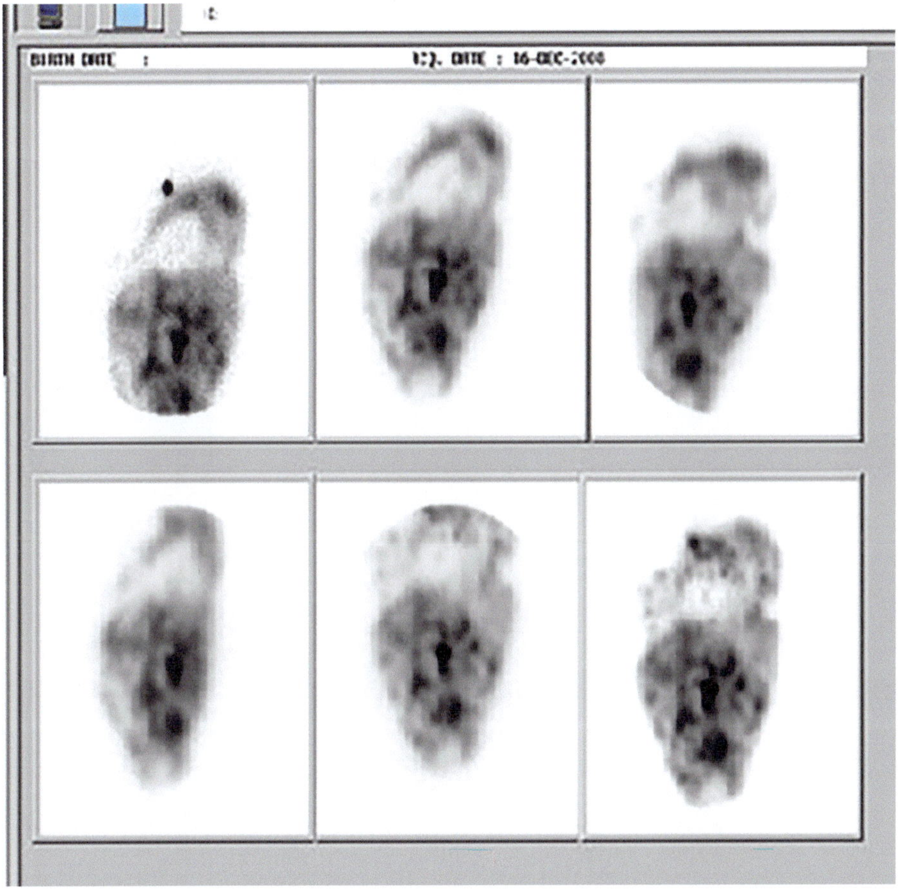

Fig. 9.2 Nonuniform distribution of dialysate fluid

ultrafiltration failure). The change from high and high average transport status to low and low average transporter status appeared due either to mild degrees of peritoneal sclerosis or lesser degrees of adhesions (Table 9.2).

In our study [12], the PD technique survival in the patients reinitiated on PD was 77.41% (24 out of 31), and patient survival was 67.72% (21 out of 31) at the end of 2 years. The technique and patient survival of the overall PD patient population were better than the reinitiated group. The technique survival was 81.3% and patient survival was 80.1% at the end of 2 years, for the overall PD population. In the previous studies [6, 8, 14], the PD technique survival after reinitiation was between 42% and 56.3%.

Table 9.1 Previous studies

	Szeto et al. [6]	Cox et al. [14]	Troidle et al. [8]	Sahu et al. [15]	Ram et al.[a] [12]
Year of publication	2002	2006	2005	2003	2014
Day on which catheter removed for refractory peritonitis	10	6.6 to 8.9	–	–	5 to 6
Number of patients reinitiated on PD	51[b]	42	88	Total reinitiations: 106; after peritonitis: 50	31[c]
Follow-up period after reinitiation of PD (months)	18.5 ± 16.8	20 ± 7.3	15.4 ± 15.4	48	24
Number of days between Tenckhoff catheter removal and reinsertion (mean)	40 days	10 ± 5.9 weeks in success group; 12 ± 7.3 weeks in failed group	–	–	50.4
Predictors of technique failure after reinitiation of PD	Severe peritonitis requiring temporary hemodialysis	Dialysis vintage	–	Increasing patient age	None identified
Outcome	At 2 years: Patient survival: 80.3% at 2 years, Technique survival: 56.3%	At the end of follow up Successful PD: 23 of 42 (54.7%), PD technique failure: 19 of 42 (45.2%)	At 12 months: On PD: 37 (42%), On PD for less than 12 months: 51 (58%)	At 48 months: continued with PD: 65 (61.3%) patients. Second catheter removed: 41 patients[d]	Patientson regular follow-up without peritonitis: 13 (41.9%), diedwhile on PD: 11 (35.4%), ultrafiltration failure: 1 (3.2%),catheter removed due to refractory peritonitis: 6 (19.3%).In the six patients in whom the catheter was removed dueto technique failure, the PD was continued for18.4 ± 9.6 months[d].

[a]See the text for further information

[b]In another 49 patients, the reinsertion failed due to intraoperative finding of peritoneal sclerosis and bowel adhesions

[c]In another 7 patients, the reinsertion failed due to intraoperative finding of bowel adhesions

[d]The study did not specify the outcomes of the patients who had second catheter placed after the removal of catheter for the peritonitis

[e]In addition, five patients had the catheter inserted for a third time, after a second episode of refractory peritonitis. The duration of PD on the third catheter was 13.2 ± 5.0 months (range 6–18)

Table 9.2 Peritoneal equilibration test

Transport category (D/P Cr reference ranges)	PET during first phase of PD ($n = 27$)	PET after reinitiation of PD ($n = 21$)	D/P Cr after reinitiation of PD (mean ± SD)
Low (0.34–0.49)	1	2	0.45 ± 0.05
Low average (0.50–0.64)	17	9	0.50 ± 0.06
High average (0.66–0.81)	9	7	0.72 ± 0.01
High (0.82–1.03)	0	3	0.88 ± 0.01

D/P Cr Dialysate plasma creatinine ratio

9.2 Conclusion

In India, 18–20% of ESKD patients opt peritoneal dialysis as their renal replacement therapy modality. PD catheter removal is often contemplated for standard indications. However, catheter reinsertion and continuation of PD do not happen successfully either due to patient or clinician's decision or preference, respectively. Evaluations to rule out peritoneal adhesions apriori and introducing the catheter either by open surgical technique or by laparoscopic insertion are associated with better outcome. A minimum of 4 weeks should elapse between the catheter removal and reinsertion. Transporter status should be evaluated periodically as it changes with reintroduction of catheter and is essential for proper PD prescription.

9.3 Important Points

- A high proportion of patients whose catheters were removed were unable to successfully reinitiate PD, due to irreversible peritoneal injury or to decisions by the patient or the nephrologist.
- A minimum of 2 to 4 weeks should be allowed between the catheter removal and reimplantation.
- Peritoneal scintigraphy and computerized tomography to be done to assess the presence of adhesions in the abdomen.
- A nonuniform distribution of the dialysate fluid, with most of it confining to the central part of the abdomen in several loculations, suggests the presence of adhesions.
- Severe peritonitis, dialysis vintage, and increasing patient age are factors that predicted the technique failure.

References

1. Reddy YNV, Abraham G, Mathew M, Ravichandran R, Reddy YNV. An Indian model for cost-effective CAPD with minimal man power and economic resources. Nephrol Dial Transplant. 2011;26:3089–91.
2. Pérez-Fontán M, Rodríguez-Carmona A. Peritoneal catheter removal for severe peritonitis: landscape after a lost battle. Perit Dial Int. 2007;27:155–8.
3. Li PK, Szeto CC, Piraino B, et al. Peritoneal dialysis-related infections recommendations: 2010 update. International society for peritoneal dialysis. Perit Dial Int. 2010;30:393–423.

4. Mitra A, Teitelbaum I. Is it safe to simultaneously remove and replace infected peritoneal dialysis catheters? Review of the literature and suggested guidelines. AdvPerit Dial. 2003;19:255–9.
5. Choi P, Nemati E, Banerjee A, Preston E, Levy J, Brown E. Peritoneal dialysis catheter removal for acute peritonitis: a retrospective analysis of factors associated with catheter removal and prolonged postoperative hospitalization. Am J Kidney Dis. 2004;43:103–11.
6. Szeto CC, Chow KM, Wong TYH, Leung CB, Wang AYM, Lui SF, Li PKT. Feasibility of resuming peritoneal dialysis after severe peritonitis and Tenckhoff catheter removal. J Am Soc Nephrol. 2002;13:1040–5.
7. Fontán PM, Rodríguez-Carmona A, García-Naveiro R, Rosales M, Villaverde P, Valdés F. Peritonitis-related mortality in patients undergoing chronic peritoneal dialysis. Perit Dial Int. 2005;25:274–84.
8. Troidle L, Gorban-Brennan N, Finkelstein FO. Outcome of patients on chronic peritoneal dialysis undergoing peritoneal catheter removal because of peritonitis. Adv Perit Dial. 2005;21:98–101.
9. Krishnan M, Thodis E, Ikonomopoulos D, et al. Predictors of outcome following bacterial peritonitis in peritoneal dialysis. Perit Dial Int. 2002;22:573–81.
10. Digenis GE, Abraham G, Savin E, et al. Peritonitis-related deaths in continuous ambulatory peritoneal dialysis patients. Perit Dial Int. 1990;10:45–7.
11. Fried LF, Bernardini J, Johnston JR, Piraino B. Peritonitis influences mortality in peritoneal dialysis patients. J Am Soc Nephrol. 1996;7:2176–82.
12. Ram R, Swarnalatha G, Dakshinamurty KV. Reinitiation of peritoneal dialysis after catheter removal for refractory peritonitis. J Nephrol. 2014 Aug;27(4):445–9.
13. Gudit S, Sudhakar P, Ram R, Prasad N, Prabhakar VV, Dakshinamurty KV. Peritoneal scintigraphy in the diagnosis of adhesions. Perit Dial Int. 2010;30:112–3.
14. Cox SD, Walsh SB, Yaqoob MM, Fan SLS. Predictors of survival and technique success after reinsertion of peritoneal dialysis catheter following severe peritonitis. Perit Dial Int. 2006;27:67–73.
15. Sahu KM, Walele A, Liakopoulos V, Bargman JM. Analysis of factors predicting survival of a second peritoneal dialysis catheter. Adv Perit Dial. 2003;19:252–4.

Peritonitis-Related Mortality

10

Gopalakrishnan Natarajan, Sheik Sulthan Alavudeen, and Shivakumar Dakshinamoorthy

Mrs. F, a 32 years old lady, with known Type 1 diabetes since the age of 9 years, was diagnosed to have advanced chronic kidney disease in 2018. She was irregular in follow-up. In July, 2022, she was initiated on continuous ambulatory peritoneal dialysis after laparoscopic placement of peritoneal catheter at a peripheral medical center. After about 2 weeks of initiation of dialysis, she developed abdominal pain and fever. There was pus discharge at the exit site and the effluent was cloudy. She presented to tertiary care kidney institute with volume overload and pulmonary oedema. Peritoneal effluent was sent for culture and she was started on hemodialysis. Intraperitoneal amikacin and vancomycin were started empirically. Culture revealed growth of *Escherichia coli*, *Staphylococcus aureus*, and filamentous fungi. Intravenous amphotericin was started.

In view of refractory peritonitis, peritoneal dialysis catheter was removed. Despite these measures, her condition deteriorated progressively and she succumbed on seventh day after admission.

10.1 Introduction

Peritonitis is a major complication of continuous ambulatory peritoneal dialysis (CAPD). Peritonitis is not only a cause of morbidity but a contributor for mortality also among patients on CAPD. However, the actual magnitude of peritonitis-related mortality (PRM) is uncertain and quite varied in different studies. The observed variations in PRM are primarily due to heterogeneity in definition of PRM and

G. Natarajan (✉) · S. S. Alavudeen · S. Dakshinamoorthy
Institute of Nephrology, Madras medical College, Chennai, India

G. Abraham et al. (eds.), *Diagnosis and Management of Complications of Peritoneal Dialysis related Peritonitis*,
https://doi.org/10.1007/978-981-99-2275-8_10

nature of population studied. When the mortality occurs during the active phase of peritonitis itself, there would not be any ambiguity in attributing peritonitis as a cause for mortality. However, classifying the deaths occurring as a sequel to the inflammatory milieu initiated and perpetuated by peritonitis as PRM is challenging. Such deaths also have to be classified as peritonitis-related mortality.

10.2 Definition

Following are few of the different definitions applied for PRM in published studies.

1. Death directly attributable to peritonitis in the clinical opinion of the treating nephrologist (Australia and New Zealand Dialysis and Transplant registry—ANZDATA) [1–4]
2. Mortality occurring i) during the course of a clinically active peritonitis, or ii) during the week after complete clinical, microbiological, and cytological remission of an episode of peritonitis, or iii) in the case of a refractory peritonitis demanding catheter removal, before hospital discharge for re-initiation of regular dialysis therapy (HD or PD) [5]
3. Mortality from any cause during antibiotic treatment (generally 2–3 weeks), depending on the organism or death during temporary hemodialysis (generally 4 weeks after catheter removal) [6]
4. Any mortality occurring within 30 days after an episode of peritonitis

This definition is more appropriate. Neil Boudville et al. [7], in an elegant case-crossover study design, analyzed the relationship between peritonitis and mortality among 1316 patients who received CAPD in Australia and New Zealand and who died while receiving CAPD or within 30 days of switching to hemodialysis. There were 1446 episodes of peritonitis. The authors studied the odds of occurrence of peritonitis during two "window periods" of 30 days each. One window period was 30 days preceding death, while the other window period was 6 months prior to death. The odds of peritonitis during the 30 days window period preceding death was sixfold higher compared to that during the window period 6 months prior to death. This observation confirms the impact of peritonitis on mortality and also provides credence to 30 days window period for the sustained negative impact of peritonitis on mortality.

In this study, out of 250 patients who had an episode of peritonitis within 30 days prior to death, only in 69 (27.6%) patients, peritonitis was the direct cause of death. The remaining patients had varied causes of death including cardiac, withdrawal, non-peritoneal infection, cerebrovascular, bowel infarction, gastrointestinal hemorrhage, and abdominal perforation.

10.3 Risk Factors for Peritonitis-Related Mortality

In a study conducted at Toronto Western Hospital, the risk factors for mortality due to peritonitis were studied. The study included 636 episodes of peritonitis which occurred in 440 patients on CAPD. There were 16 deaths. The three risk factors identified were (1) infection with *Staphylococcus aureus* and multiple microbes, (2) delayed removal of peritoneal catheter, and (3) preexisting cardiovascular disease [8].

In an Indian study, the authors observed that patients with hypertension, diabetes, and left ventricular dysfunction had higher peritonitis-related mortality [9].

Most of the studies have revealed a higher risk for mortality in patients with peritonitis due to *Staphylococcus aureus*, fungi, and multiple microbes.

Delayed presentation of patients (as in the case scenario described above) and delayed removal of peritoneal dialysis catheter in refractory peritonitis are important predisposing factors for mortality.

Old age, female gender, malnutrition, and depression have been identified as correlates of increased mortality associated with peritonitis [5].

Hongjian Ye et al. [10] studied the impact of duration of peritoneal dialysis therapy on peritonitis-related mortality. The study involved 1321 patients on CAPD for a median period of 31 months. It was observed that peritonitis strongly influenced mortality in patients who were on CAPD for longer than 2 years.

In a recent study of mortality trends after transfer from peritoneal dialysis to hemodialysis, a higher risk for mortality was observed during the first 30 days of transfer. This study incorporated data of 4 registries covering 21 countries. Old age, longer peritoneal dialysis vintage, and transfer due to peritonitis were associated with increased mortality [11].

10.4 Causes for Peritonitis-Related Mortality

The following are the common causes for peritonitis-related mortality reported in the literature:

1. Peritonitis leading into sepsis
2. Cardiovascular death (myocardial infarction, cardiac failure)
3. Cerebrovascular events
4. Non-peritoneal infections
5. Perforation of abdominal viscus
6. Bowel infarction

10.5 Peritonitis and Cardiovascular Mortality

An analysis of BRAZPD II cohort (Brazilian national study) between 2004 and 2011 revealed a 22% increased risk of cardiovascular mortality associated with peritonitis and the risk increased progressively with additional episodes of peritonitis [12].

Hicham Cheikh Hassan et al. [13], in a longitudinal observational cohort study using Australia and New Zealand Peritoneal Dialysis Registry (ANZDATA), analyzed the data pertaining to 9699 patients who received CAPD. There were 8936 peritonitis episodes in 4353 patients. Cardiovascular death (myocardial infarction, cardiac failure, cerebrovascular event, rupture of aortic aneurysm) occurred in 1405 patients. Cardiovascular mortality was more common among patients who experienced peritonitis episode than in those who did not have peritonitis (58.2 vs 33.5 per 1000 patient years, $P < 0.001$). Even a single episode of peritonitis was associated with heightened risk of cardiovascular mortality (adjusted HR [aHR] 1.31, 95% CI 1.17–1.47, $P < 0.001$), and the risk progressively increased with more number of peritonitis episodes.

The pathomechanism of increased cardiovascular mortality risk imposed by peritonitis is hypothesized to be due to inflammation. Chronic kidney disease is a state of heightened inflammation. There are additional cardiovascular risk factors in CAPD patients, viz. hyperlipidemia, exposure to glucose, and weight gain. Peritonitis episode elicits local and systemic inflammation adding onto total inflammatory burden. The additional acute inflammatory burden confers short-term as well as long-term cardiovascular disease and mortality risk.

10.6 Prevention of Peritonitis-Related Mortality

The important strategies to prevent PRM comprise of prevention of peritonitis, early diagnosis of peritonitis, and initiation of appropriate antimicrobial therapy for peritonitis [14]:

1. Strict adherence to the International Society of Peritoneal Dialysis guidelines with regard to prevention of peritonitis has to be ensured.
2. Appropriate training, prophylactic antibiotics prior to colonoscopy and invasive gynecological procedures, correction of hypokalemia, avoidance of use of H2 receptor antagonists, and administration of prophylactic antifungal agent during antibiotic therapy are some of the preventive measures of peritonitis.
3. Education of patients on the signs and symptoms of peritonitis and sensitization on the importance of early reporting to hospital are of paramount importance.
4. Ensuring appropriate techniques for culture of peritoneal effluent and rapid identification of the causative organism are of immense value.
5. Early initiation of empiric antimicrobial therapy as per the guidelines has to be ensured.

6. Removal of peritoneal dialysis catheter without delay in patients with refractory peritonitis is mandatory.
7. Identification of cardiovascular risk factors, viz., hypertension, diabetes, dyslipidemia, and smoking and optimizing their control are of immense value.

10.7 Important Points

- Peritonitis is a significant contributor for morbidity and mortality among patients on CAPD therapy.
- Peritonitis-related mortality refers to any death occurring within 30 days after an episode of peritonitis.
- Sepsis and cardiovascular events are the major causes for peritonitis-related mortality.
- Staphylococcal peritonitis, fungal peritonitis, and polymicrobial peritonitis are associated with increased risk for mortality.
- Delayed removal of peritoneal dialysis catheter in refractory peritonitis portends a high risk for mortality.
- Strict observance of preventive measures for peritonitis and optimization of control and management of cardiovascular risk factors are of paramount importance.

References

1. Barraclough K, Hawley CM, McDonald SP, Brown FG, Rosman JB, Wiggins KJ, Bannister KM, Johnson DW. Polymicrobial peritonitis in peritoneal dialysis patients in Australia: predictors, treatment, and outcomes. Am J Kidney Dis. 2010;14(55):121–31.
2. Burke M, Hawley CM, Badve SV, McDonald SP, Brown FG, Boudville N, Wiggins KJ, Bannister KM, Johnson DW. Relapsing and recurrent peritoneal dialysis-associated peritonitis: a multicenter registry study. Am J Kidney Dis. 2011;15(58):429–36.
3. Edey M, Hawley CM, McDonald SP, Brown FG, Rosman JB, Wiggins KJ, Bannister KM, Johnson DW. Enterococcal peritonitis in Australian peritoneal dialysis patients: predictors, treatment and outcomes in 116 cases. Nephrol Dial Transplant. 2010;16(25):1272–8.
4. Fahim M, Hawley CM, McDonald SP, Brown FG, Rosman JB, Wiggins KJ, Bannister KM, Johnson DW. Culture-negative peritonitis in peritoneal dialysis patients in Australia: predictors, treatment, and outcomes in 435 cases. Am J Kidney Dis. 2010;17(55):690–7.
5. Pérez-Fontan M, Rodríguez-Carmona A, García-Naveiro R, Rosales M, Villaverde P, Valdés F. Peritonitis-related mortality in patients undergoing chronic peritoneal dialysis. Perit Dial Int. 2005;25:274–84.
6. Szeto CC, Kwan BC, Chow KM, Law MC, Pang WF, Leung CB, Li PK. Repeat peritonitis in peritoneal dialysis: retrospective review of 181 consecutive cases. Clin J Am Soc Nephrol. 2011;24(6):827–33.
7. Boudville N, Kemp A, Clayton P, Lim W, Badve SV, Hawley CM, McDonald SP, Wiggins KJ, Bannister KM, Brown FG, Johnson DW. Recent peritonitis associates with mortality among patients treated with peritoneal dialysis. J Am Soc Nephrol. 2012;23:1398–405. https://doi.org/10.1681/ASN.201112113.

8. George E. Digenis, Georgi Abraham, et al, peritonitis-related deaths in continuous ambulatory peritoneal dialysis (CAPD) patients. Perit Dial Int. 1990;10:45–7.
9. Krishnaprasad D, Reddy YNV, Rohit A, Varma A, Mathew M, Revathy L, Nair S, Abraham G. Peritonitis-related deat–a retrospective studyanalysing causative factors in chronic peritoneal dialysis. Ind J Perit Dial. 2013;24:274.
10. Ye H, Zhou Q, Fan L, et al. The impact of peritoneal dialysis-related peritonitis on mortality in peritoneal dialysis patients. BMC Nephrol. 2017;18:186.
11. Nadeau-Fredette AC, Sukul N, Lambie M, et al. Mortality trends after transfer from peritoneal dialysis to hemodialysis. Kidney Int Rep. 2022;7:1062–73.
12. Pecoits-Filho R, Yabumoto FM, Campos LG, Moraes TP, Figueiredo AE, Olandoski M, et al. Peritonitis as a risk factor for long-term cardiovascular mortality in peritoneal dialysis patients: the case of a friendly fire? Nephrology (Carlton). 2018;23(3):253–8.
13. Cheikh Hassan HI, Murali K, Lonergan M, Boudville N, Johnson D, Borlace M, Chen JH. Association of Peritonitis with cardiovascular mortality over time in the peritoneal dialysis population, an ANZDATA registry study. Kidney International Reports. 2022;7:2388. https://doi.org/10.1016/j.ekir.2022.08.008.
14. ISPD Peritonitis guideline recommendations. 2022 update on prevention and treatment. Perit Dial Int. 2022;42(2):110–53.

11 Indications and Findings on Peritoneal Biopsy

Anil Tarigopula, Yuvaram Reddy, N. V. Seethalekshmy, and Georgi Abraham

11.1 Recurrent Hemoperitoneum

A 68-year-old lady with CKD stage 5 following recent COVID was initiated on hemodialysis. She developed recurrent access thrombosis and hence was switched to CAPD with 3 exchanges of 2 L dextrose containing fluid. While implanting the swan neck catheter in July 2021, biopsy of peritoneum showed no significant changes. As her lung imaging showed lung parenchymal cavitating and non-cavitating lesions and multiple mediastinal lymph nodes, with positive Mantoux test and hypoxemia, a presumptive diagnosis of tuberculosis was made. She was empirically initiated on four drug antituberculous treatment in August 2021. The visualized upper abdominal sections and extension of CT chest to abdomen showed multiple retroperitoneal enlarged lymph nodes with signs of caseation. She continued on CAPD with good quality of life while on four drug antituberculous therapy which was continued for 6 months. From 9.03.2022 onwards, the dialysis effluent was hemorrhagic; she was not on aspirin/clopidogrel or any anticoagulants. Her prothrombin time and coagulation profile were normal. Despite clearing up of hemoperitoneum with repeated flushing using intraperitoneal heparin, the hemoperitoneum continued with fall in hematocrit. CT abdomen with contrast was done

A. Tarigopula · G. Abraham (✉)
MGM Healthcare, Chennai, Tamil Nadu, India

Y. Reddy
University of Pennsylvania, Philadelphia, USA

N. V. Seethalekshmy
Amrita Institute of Medical Science Kochi, Kochi, Kerala, India

G. Abraham et al. (eds.), *Diagnosis and Management of Complications of Peritoneal Dialysis related Peritonitis*,
https://doi.org/10.1007/978-981-99-2275-8_11

which showed multiple hypodense, poorly enhancing lesions, replacing the entire myometrium of uterus, and multiple hypodense lesions in the liver, pancreas, and peritoneum. The hemorrhagic dialysis effluent culture grew gram-negative bacilli. CEA was 6.5 mg/l, just above the normal range. A laparoscopic examination of the peritoneal cavity showed multiple nodular lesions in both lobes of the liver and peritoneum which were oozing blood. Peritoneal biopsy showed metastatic adenocarcinoma with areas of necrosis. Other investigations of the patient were unremarkable. CAPD was discontinued, catheter was removed, and the patient transferred permanently to hemodialysis through a jugular access [1, 2]. As she was frail with a weight of 38 kgs and had metastatic adenocarcinoma, the poor prognosis was explained to the patient and family. There was progressive fall in blood pressures, and within a short while of shifting to hemodialysis, she died at home. We present the report of a lady with pulmonary tuberculosis treated successfully who developed metastatic adenocarcinoma of the abdominal cavity leading to recurrent hemoperitoneum, diagnosed using a peritoneal biopsy (Figs. 11.1 and 11.2).

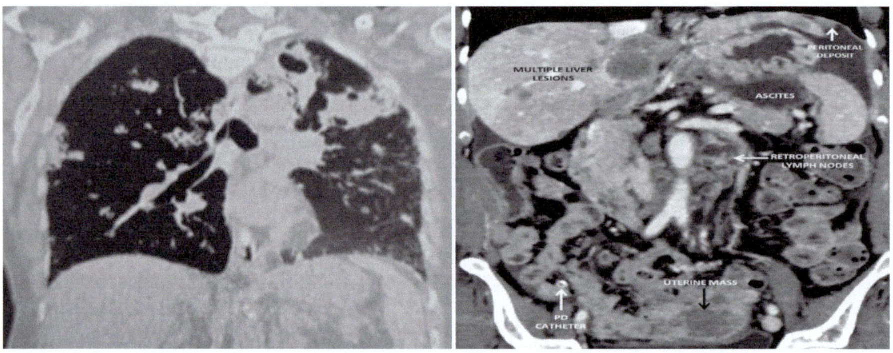

Fig. 11.1 CT of the chest and abdomen showing cavitatory and non-cavitatory lung lesions and multiple hypodense metastatic lesions in the abdominal viscera

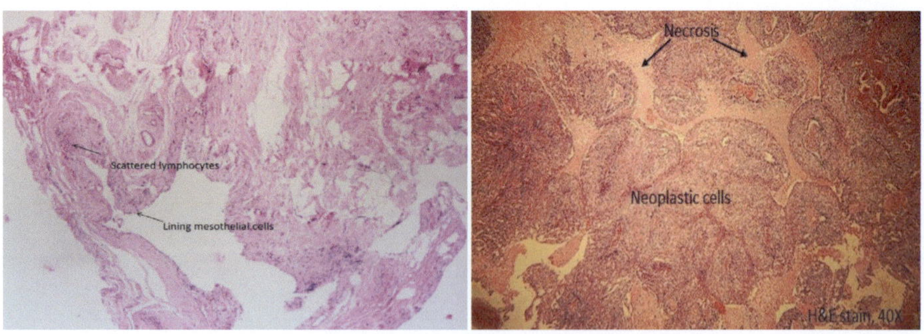

Fig. 11.2 Histological picture of peritoneum without and with adenocarcinoma

11.2 Primary Membrane Failure

An 87 years old male patient with ESKD and Waldenström macroglobulinemia had a Georgi and Sathish swan neck double cuff peritoneal dialysis catheter percutaneously implanted under local anesthesia. After a break-in period of 2 weeks, he was initiated on CAPD 2 L dianeal 3 exchanges of 2 L dextrose containing fluid. There was no ultrafiltration and he continued to have weight gain. The dialysis dwell time was shortened to obtain increased ultrafiltration using higher concentration of dextrose containing fluid. Despite this, he developed fluid overload. Icodextrin was tried along with dextrose containing fluid. The patient had no ultrafiltration and absorbed dialysis fluid. There was no evidence of any extraperitoneal leak. Peritoneal dialysis was discontinued for 2 weeks to give rest to the peritoneum while maintaining the patient on hemodialysis. Repeated attempts at PD failed and the catheter were removed and patient continued on hemodialysis. A peritoneal biopsy done at the time of catheter removal showed extensive fibrosis of the peritoneum. The patient had no previous peritonitis or abdominal surgery (Fig. 11.3).

A 60 years old male with diabetic kidney disease and IgA nephropathy underwent PD catheter implantation with a swan neck Tenckhoff double cuff catheter. He had no previous history of peritonitis or abdominal surgery. After break-in period of 2 weeks, he was initiated on CAPD with 2 L dextrose containing fluid 3–4 times a day. He did not have any ultrafiltration in spite of giving rest to the peritoneum on 2 occasions spanning 1–2 weeks. He was switched over to hemodialysis, and catheter was removed and a peritoneal biopsy was done at that time (Fig. 11.4). The peritoneal biopsy showed fibrosis and foreign body granuloma formation.

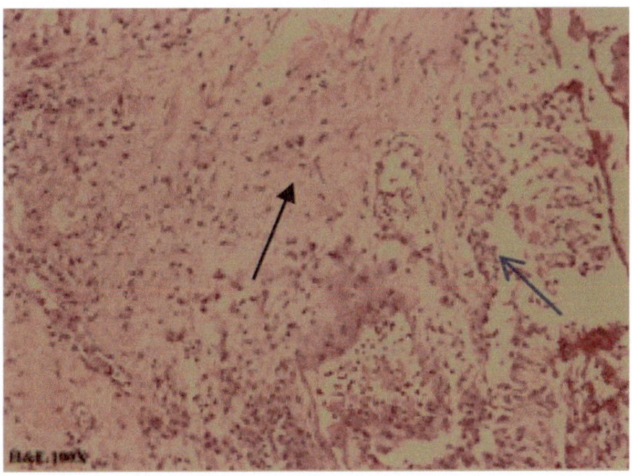

Fig. 11.3 Peritoneal biopsy showing extensive fibrosis with neovascularization thin wall vessels (white arrow) mesothelial lining (black arrow). Masson's trichrome staining of peritoneal biopsy showing fibrosis (yellow arrow)

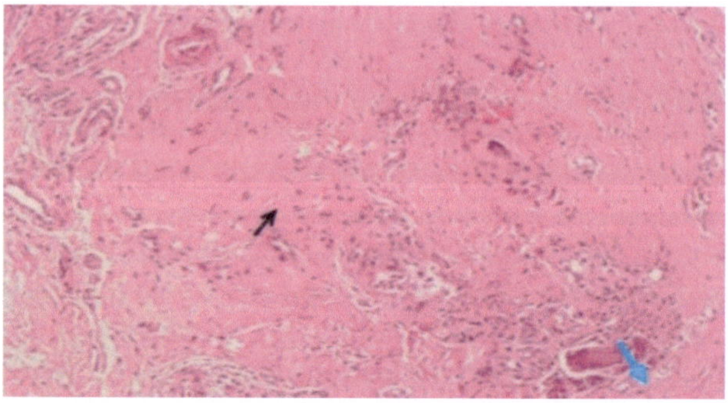

Fig. 11.4 Hematoxylin and eosin staining of peritoneal biopsy demonstrating fibrosis (black arrow) and foreign body granuloma (blue arrow)

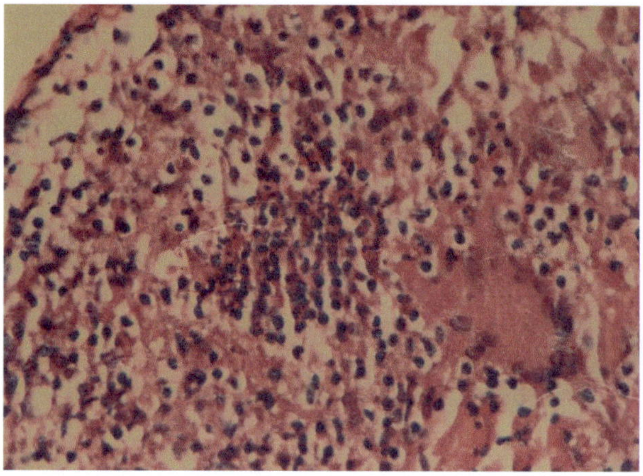

Fig. 11.5 Granulomatous inflammation of peritoneum with Langhans type giant cells and lymphocytic infiltration suggesting the possibility of mycobacterial tuberculosis infection

11.3 Peritoneal Tuberculosis

A 55-year-old lady with diabetic kidney disease and heart disease had a swan neck Tenckhoff double cuff catheter implanted, and a peritoneal biopsy was taken. She was running low grade fever with mild ascites. Peritoneal biopsy showed epithelioid granuloma with Langhans type giant cells. A chest X-ray showed right apical lesion suggestive of mycobacterium tuberculosis infection although sputum was negative for AFB smear. Mantoux test was strongly positive. She was started on quadruple antituberculous drugs which included isoniazid, rifampicin, pyrazinamide, and levofloxacin. She continued on this and her fever resolved. PD was not initiated. Two weeks later, she had a myocardial infraction and died. Peritoneal biopsy shown in Fig. 11.5 shows granulomatous inflammation with Langhans type giant cells and lymphocytic infiltration suggesting tuberculosis [3].

11.4 Sclerosing Peritonitis

A 65-year-old lady with diabetes kidney disease on CAPD for 2 years with 2.5% 2 L dextrose containing fluid four exchanges a day was a low average transporter. She had an episode of *Staphylococcus aureus* peritonitis at the start of CAPD that was satisfactorily treated.

She presented with dialysis effluent outflow obstruction of 3 days duration. X-ray abdomen showed tip of the catheter abutting the bony pelvis. There was no evidence of an extraperitoneal leak. Through a mini laparotomy, catheter was repositioned with no beneficial effect, with removal of extensive adhesions in the pelvic cavity. Peritoneal biopsy showed fibrocollagenous connective tissue containing dense infiltration of plasma cells, lymphocytes, and neutrophils. Light microscopic diagnosis was focal necrosis with subacute chronic inflammation (Fig. 11.6). Electron microscopic findings were interstitial fibrosis, thickened and laminated capillary basement membrane, thickened peritoneal lining membrane, increased fibroblasts, and macrophages in the interstitial space, consistent with chronic fibrosing peritoneal disease [4–6] (Fig. 11.7).

After reinitiating peritoneal dialysis, there was hemoperitoneum and issues with ultrafiltration, and she was continued on intermittent hemodialysis. However. as in our previous experience, rest to peritoneum may change the transport characteristics for enabling better solute transport and ultrafiltration (Fig. 11.8).

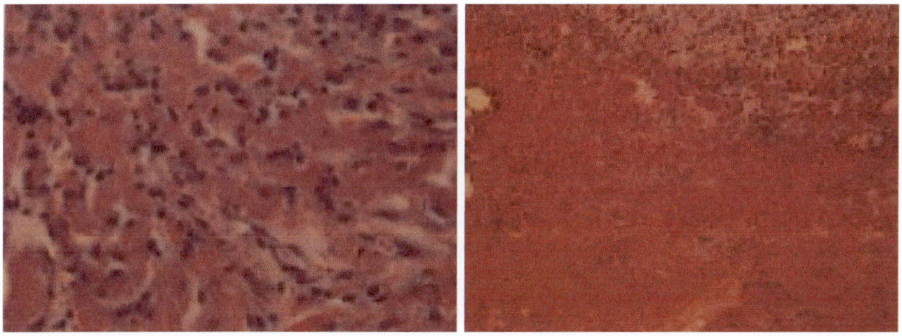

Fig. 11.6 Lymphocytes, plasma cells neutrophils, necrosis, and hemorrhage

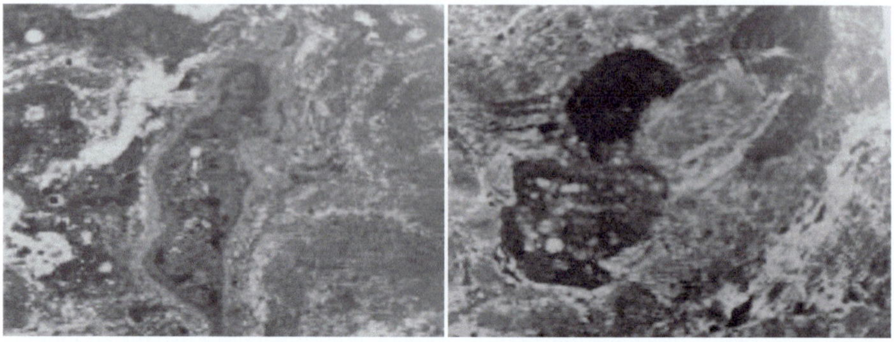

Fig. 11.7 Interstitial fibrosis, thickened and laminated capillary basement membrane. Thickened peritoneal lining membrane

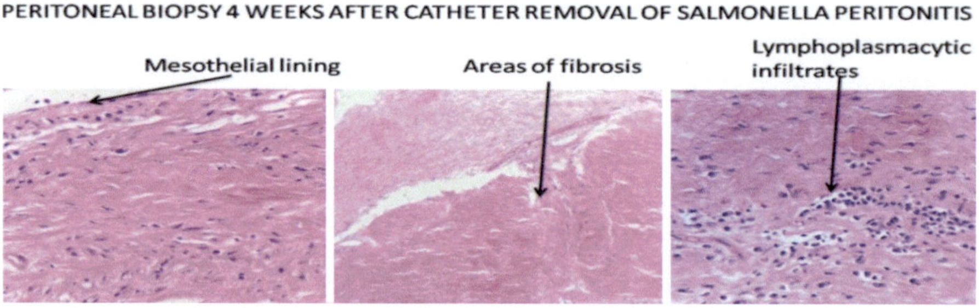

Fig. 11.8 Peritoneal biopsy 4 weeks after salmonella peritonitis necessitating catheter removal

11.5 Discussion

The peritoneal cavity is lined by a serous membrane derived from the mesoderm and is composed of single layer of mesothelial cells resting on a basement membrane, and submesothelial area has blood vessels, fibroblast, and lymphatics. A thin layer of peritoneal fluid separates the parietal and visceral mesothelial which are supported by a fibrous submesothelial layer of connective tissue. This peritoneum is a nearly continuous membrane lining the potential space between intra-abdominal viscera and abdominal wall. That total surface area of the peritoneum is approximately 1–2 m^2. Diaphragmatic peritoneum has the greater part of the parietal peritoneum and is predominantly responsible for functional peritoneal dialysis [7].

Of the serous membranes, the peritoneum has high complexity with the parietal layer covering the abdominal wall, diaphragm, anterior surfaces of retroperitoneal viscera, and pelvis. The visceral peritoneum invests the intestine and other intra-abdominal viscera. The peritoneum also covers the mesentery which contains blood vessels, lymphatics, lymph nodes, and nerves. The greater omentum is a double sheet with focal areas of mesothelium between which there are blood vessels in adipose tissue and lymphatics and lymph nodes are prominent and in the mesentery.

The peritoneal cavity is grossly divided into the greater sac over the intestines, the retrogastric lesser sac, the right and left retrocolic areas, and the pelvis. The peritoneal membrane has variably distributed stomata which are deep gaps in between adjacent cuboidal mesothelial cells, covered at some places by the microvilli on the surface of mesothelial cells. These stomata communicate with submesothelial connective tissue with a rich plexus of lymphatics that carry away peritoneal fluid and particles. Milky spots on the peritoneum and on the omentum are described as glomerular capillary network of blood vessels, which enable fluid exchange between the renal cavity, blood stream, and surrounding omental tissue. These lie directly beneath the stomata and are associated with macrophages, T and B lymphocytes, and plasma cells. Peritoneal membrane serves as a selective barrier for fluid and cells.

In a *normal peritoneal tissue*, cross section of normal mesothelial cells shows these cells to be thin and flattened on histology sections. However, exfoliated sheets of normal mesothelial cells may be evident in cytology preparations of peritoneal washes taken during a laparotomy. These cells on microscopy appear to have abundant clear cytoplasm with well-defined cell borders and small, centrally placed nuclei with homogeneous chromatin pattern and usually do not have a prominent nucleolus. The submesothelial layer normally contains few cells, mostly fibroblasts.

Reactive mesothelium occurs in a variety of reactive processes, and the mesothelial cells undergo markedly proliferative and hyperplastic changes. In reactive processes, the relatively abundant cytoplasm is maintained, but the cell borders become less well defined. Nuclei are usually enlarged, both absolutely and relatively. Chromatin appears dense and hyperchromatic; nucleoli become prominent. With clustering of reactive mesothelial cells, the outer border of mesothelium appears irregular. Cytoplasm appears multivacuolated and the cells may be degenerated and imbibe fluid. During reactive processes, the submesothelial layer becomes more prominent as myofibroblasts, inflammatory cells, and capillaries proliferate in this layer.

Patients on prolonged peritoneal dialysis may have *progressive morphological changes which include deterioration of peritoneal membranes*. This can be evaluated by performing serial peritoneal membrane biopsies, before peritoneal dialysis catheter insertion and catheter removal when mandated. Peritoneal biopsy is usually taken from the parietal peritoneum, at a point away from the insertion site of peritoneal dialysis catheter to avoid histologic artefacts. Biopsies are taken in a manner to prevent distortion and shrinkage of the peritoneum and avoiding electrocautery artefacts. Specimens are usually collected at room temperature in 10% neutral buffered formalin; 3–4 μm sections are cut, stained with hematoxylin and mucin, mass, and trichrome and one lesion stain.

Morphological changes indicative of *deteriorative changes in the peritoneal membrane* include (1) denudation of mesothelial cells, (2) thickening and sclerotic changes in submesothelial connective tissue, (3) vasculopathy, (4) angiogenesis, and (5) neomembrane formation on the existing peritoneum. The thickness of submesothelial connective tissue is usually indicative of the thickness of so-called submesothelial compact zone (SCZ), immediately below the mesothelial cell layer up to the deep fatty tissue layer. Vasculopathy is evaluated by measuring the thickness of post capillary venules which have a normal size of 25–50 μm. Parameters used to evaluate vasculopathy include vascular wall thickening and vascular lumen stenosis and ratio of luminal diameter to the vessel external diameter (L/V ratio). Angiogenesis is diagnosed by looking at microvascular density per unit of tissue area on light microscopy.

Typically, normal peritoneum shows intact mesothelial cells on the surface with preservation of submesothelial compact zone and the deep fatty layer with no evidence of distortion or shrinkage. Peritoneal biopsies from patient's diagnosed with *encapsulated peritoneal sclerosis* show mesothelial cell denudation, marked thickening of submesothelial compact zone (SCC) with collagenous tissue degeneration, thickened blood vessels with luminal obliteration of capillaries, and post capillary venules and in some cases arteriolar calcification.

Peritoneal biopsy may also be performed in patients on peritoneal dialysis presenting with ascites, with clinical suspicion of infective peritonitis. In cases of bacterial peritonitis, microscopic features of chronic inflammation with lymphocytes and plasma cells may be observed. Cases with active peritoneal tuberculosis can show epithelioid granulomatous inflammation with Langhans type giant cells with without necrosis. In case of fungal peritonitis, evaluation of peritoneal biopsy may show fungal organisms. In cases with malignant ascites, evaluation of peritoneal biopsy may reveal tumor deposits [8]. Additional microbiological culture and molecular studies are required for confirmation of etiologic diagnosis.

Histologic assessment of peritoneal tissue using appropriately collected peritoneal biopsy samples is necessary for evaluation of presence and extent of peritoneal damage caused by peritoneal dialysis and for diagnosis of encapsulated peritoneal sclerosis. In some cases with ascites and clinically suspected peritonitis, peritoneal biopsy may show morphologic features pointing to an inflammatory or infectious etiology.

The primary objective of peritoneal dialysis is solute removal (uremic toxins) and excess fluid removal (ultrafiltration). The peritoneal membrane characteristics change after peritonitis with low transporter and low average transporter status changing to high average and high transporter status due to neovascularization and peritoneal fibrosis. However, the development of dysregulation of solute transport and ultrafiltration problem may be temporary and gets better over a period of time unless it is due to mycobacterium tuberculosis infection, fungal peritonitis, or coinfections of *Pseudomonas aeruginosa* and *Staphylococcus aureus* peritonitis. Under these circumstances, secondary failure of the peritoneum will lead to switch over to hemodialysis. The above illustration are a few examples of the usefulness of peritoneal biopsy in deciding the continuation of peritoneal dialysis using either CAPD or APD in high transporters. In primary peritoneal membrane failure with no previous history of Peritoneal TB after sentence endind with infiltration, abdominal surgery is a very infrequent occurrence as demonstrated above. A genetic study of peritoneal tissue may be useful along with proteomics and metabolomics in primary peritoneal membrane failure.

A study of peritoneal biopsies by our group did not find a direct correlation between peritoneal scarring and ultrafiltration volume. This may have been due to sampling error. If permanent PD catheter implantation is done under laparoscopic guidance, a good look at peritoneum and taking multiple biopsy specimens with light microscopy and electron microscopic examination can yield important histological information.

A Correlative Study of Peritoneal Biopsy Depicting Fibrosis as a Marker of Ultrafiltration and Solute Transport

A prospective study was undertaken to look at peritoneal fibrosis and various other parameters including severity of peritoneal fibrosis and DKD patients and those without DKD (Fig. 11.9).

Scatterplot of ultrafiltration per day and percentage of peritoneal fibrosis in 26 patients studied was not statistically significant with p value of ($P = 0.0830$).

Between diabetics and non-diabetics, the T-test of peritoneal fibrosis mean score was 65,000 and 65,400, respectively, with P value of (0.974) (Fig. 11.10).

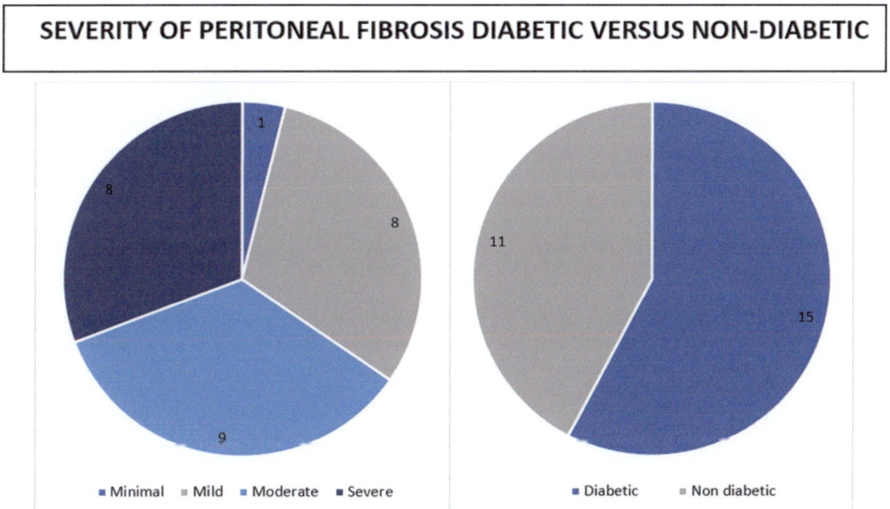

Fig. 11.9 Distribution of patients according to severity of the PF ($N = 26$), prevalence of DM

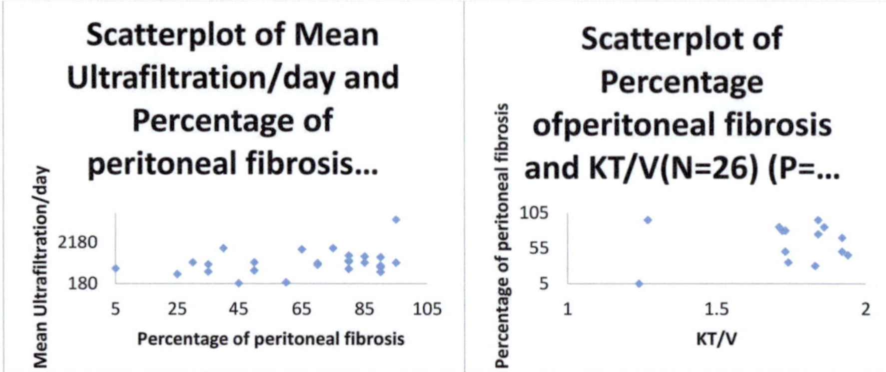

Fig. 11.10 Showing scatterplots of UF and KT/V

11.6 Important Points

- Peritoneal biopsy either at the time of catheter implantation or catheter removal is easy to perform.
- Following an episode of peritonitis histomorphometry of the peritoneum will provide important information which can be correlated with peritoneal membrane function such as transport status.
- Sampling issues may be a deterrent as peritoneal surface area is 1–2 m^2; hence, important findings may be missed.
- We did not find a direct correlation between ultrafiltration, solute transport, and peritoneal fibrosis on biopsy.
- Biopsy findings especially mycobacterium tuberculosis peritonitis, neoplastic lesions, and primary and secondary membrane failure are evident on microscopic examination in tailoring treatment strategies.

References

1. Hendricks PMEM, et al. Peritoneal sclerosis in continuous peritoneal dialysis patients: analysis of clinical presentation, risk factors and peritoneal transport kinetics. Perit Dial Int. 1997;17:136–43.
2. Rottembourg J, et al. Severe abdominal complications in patients undergoing CAPD. Eur Dial Int 1997: Transplant Assoc Proc. 1983;20:231–42.
3. Rohit A, Abraham G. Peritoneal dialysis related peritonitis due to Mycobacterium spp.: a case report and review of literature. J Epidemiol Glob Health. 2016;6:243–8.
4. Ingg T, et al. Peritoneal sclerosis in peritoneal dialysis patients. Am J Nephrol. 1984;4:173–6.
5. Korzets A, et al. Sclerosing peritonitis. Possible easily diagnosis by CT of the abdomen. Am J Nephrol. 1988;8:143–6.

6. Krestin GP, et al. Imaging diagnosis of sclerosing peritonitis and relation of radiological signs to the extent of the disease. Abdom Imaging. 1995;20:414–20.
7. Ghosh S, Yuvaraj A, Vijayan M, Raghava MR, Abraham Revathi L, Nair S. A correlative study of peritoneal biopsy depicting fibrosis as a marker of ultrafiltration and solute transport. Ind J Perit Dial. 2015;28:23–6.
8. Liu Y-H, Ma H-X, Ji B, Coa D-B. Spontaneous hemoperitoneum from hepatic metastatic trophoblastic tumor. World J Gastroenterol. 2012 Aug 21;18(31):4237–40.

Usefulness of Imaging of PD-Related Complications

12

Priya Masilamani, Chandrasekaran Venkatraman, Subramanian Jeyaraj, and Georgi Abraham

Clinical Vignettes

1. 54 years old male, with diabetes mellitus and severe LV dysfunction, on CAPD, presented to another hospital with dialysate outflow block. The plain x-ray picture showed the catheter tip migration to the left lumbar region (Fig. 12.1b). This migration of a swan neck catheter can happen either due to omental trapping or constipation (Fig. 12.1a). He had abdominal pain and rebound tenderness suggestive of peritonitis. The nephrologist elsewhere thought that the outflow block was due to fibrin clot in the intraperitoneal part of the catheter. Intraperitoneal streptokinase 7.5lakh units were instilled through the catheter with no beneficial effect. This led to intraperitoneal bleeding and drop in hemoglobin. Patient presented to us after 48 h with hyperkalemia, acute abdomen, and severe anemia. Before we could remove the catheter, patient succumbed to sepsis and intraperitoneal hemorrhage. Treatment for constipation is use of laxatives, proctoclysis enema, or soap and water enema.
2. 54 years old lady, on CAPD for 17 years, had peritonitis due to gram-positive organism and was treated with intraperitoneal antibiotics. She suffered from TB peritonitis 15 years ago which was successfully treated for 18 months leading to complete resolution. She is anuric. She underwent a parathyroidectomy for tertiary hyperparathyroidism 4 years ago: serum creatinine 6.44 mg/dl, albumin 3.49 gm/dl, Hb 12.1gm/dl, WBC count 7600cells/cu.mm., platelet count 269000cells/cu.mm., ESR 42 mm/hr., i PTH 129 pg/ml, glucose 138 mg/dl 2 h postprandial, serum calcium 8.4 mg/dl, serum phosphorus 4.2 mg/dl

P. Masilamani (✉) · C. Venkatraman · G. Abraham
MGM Healthcare, Chennai, Tamil Nadu, India

S. Jeyaraj
Jeyanth Nallathambi Hospital, Tuticorin, Tamil Nadu, India

G. Abraham et al. (eds.), *Diagnosis and Management of Complications of Peritoneal Dialysis related Peritonitis*,
https://doi.org/10.1007/978-981-99-2275-8_12

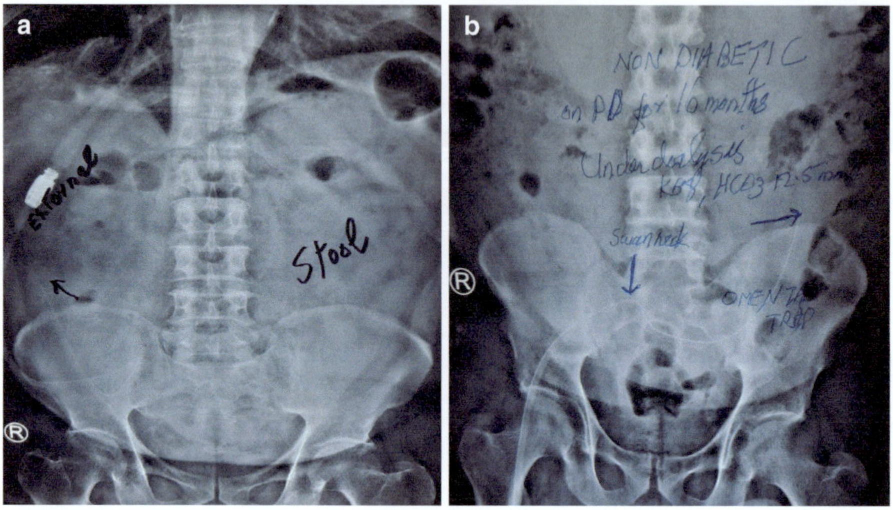

Fig. 12.1 (**a**) X-ray abdomen migrated catheter tip in the right lumbar region due to constipation. (**b**) X-ray abdomen shows migrated catheter tip in left lumbar region

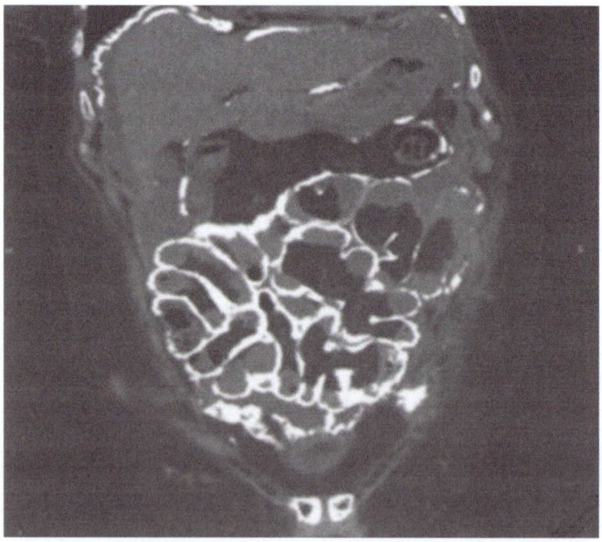

Fig. 12.2 CT showing diffuse linear calcifications in parietal and visceral peritoneum

As she had low ultrafiltration, a CT scan of the abdomen was done (Fig. 12.2), which showed linear calcifications in the peritoneum. As this was an unexpected finding, patient was switched over to icodextrin 7.5% 2 L one exchange along with three exchanges of dextrose. She is doing well in terms of ultrafiltration, solute removal, and physical well-being. Eighteen months later, she is doing well on CAPD.

3. 46 years old nondiabetic lady who had *Pseudomonas aeruginosa* peritonitis leading to catheter removal. She underwent intermittent hemodialysis and reimplantation of a Georgi and Sathish swan neck permanent PD catheter. Two weeks later, CAPD was reinitiated using two liters of dextrose containing fluid. There was minimal leak at the exit site. Dialysis was stopped. Twelve days later, she was initiated on CAPD. The ultrasound imaging of the tunnel shows no pericatheter collection/fluid ensuring that there is no further leak (Fig. 12.3). Catheter tunnel ultrasound should be done regularly in the diagnosis of catheter tunnel infections and in instances of suspected pericatheter leak. This will help in either stopping the peritoneal dialysis temporarily when pericatheter leak is there or continuing PD when no evidence of pericatheter leak is there. An ultrasound examination of the tunnel with the absence of pericatheter fluid collection rules out major leaks and tunnel infection.
4. A 77-year-old male diabetic with end-stage kidney disease was implanted a Georgi and Sathish swan neck catheter. During the flushing of the catheter, he experienced abdominal pain in the right iliac fossa. He was treated with soap and water enema for constipation. Dialysis effluent grew gram-negative organism. A CT scan of the abdomen showed large mucocele of the appendix (Fig. 12.4) with probable microperforations and peritonitis necessitating removal of catheter and switch over to hemodialysis.
5. 56 years old male nondiabetic CKD-Stage 5 was started on CAPD in 2017 May. He was using 1.5% dextrose two liters three times a day. In June 2018, he presented with progressive swelling in the left paraumbilical area which on examination showed 5x5cm nontender swelling. CT scan of the abdomen showed a collection in left paraumbilical region extending up to the left hypochondrium causing a mass effect on bowel loops (Fig. 12.5). A diagnosis of abdominal pseudocyst was made though he had no episodes of peritonitis. Patient was switched over to hemodialysis and pseudocyst resolved by itself. As the peritoneal fluid encircles the tip of the catheter in the form of a cyst, catheter dysfunction can occur. Fluid in the cyst is peritoneal dialysate. Management is surgical with resection of cyst and removal of the peritoneal dialysis catheter.

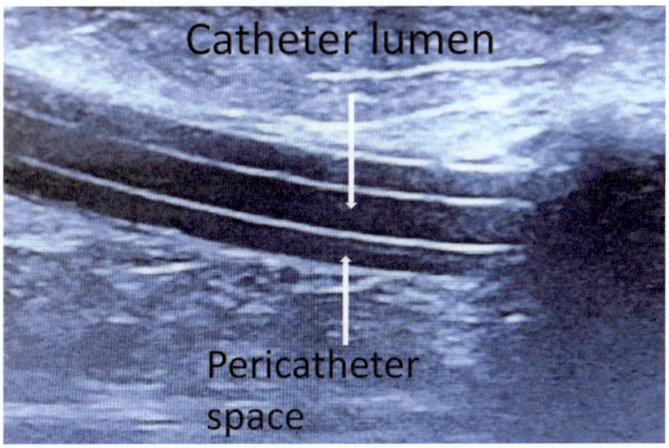

Fig. 12.3 Ultrasound picture of a normal catheter tunnel

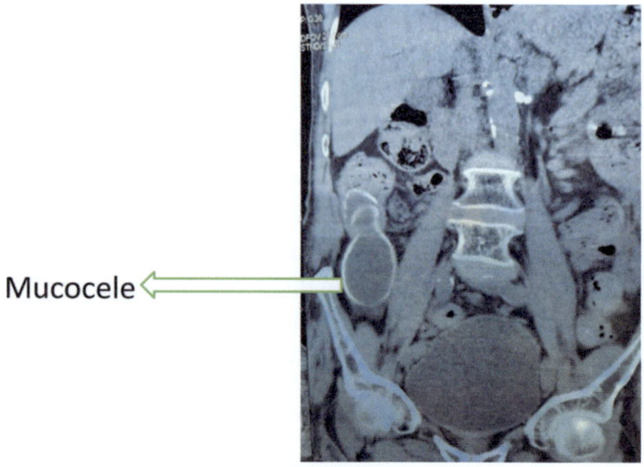

Fig. 12.4 CT showing mucocele of appendix

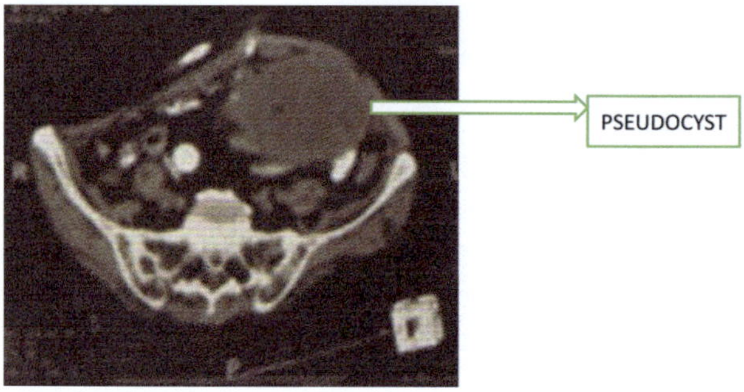

Fig. 12.5 Axial section of CT showing large paraumbilical cyst compressing on the bowel loops

6. A 33 years old lady with end-stage kidney disease secondary to SLE on hemodialysis for 3 years presented with congestive heart failure due to rheumatic mitral and tricuspid regurgitation. Hemoperitoneum was noticed while implanting a Swan neck Tenckhoff catheter. A contrast CT showed splenic infarction and capsular breach (Fig. 12.6). Ascites turned out to be positive for mycobacterium tuberculosis by PCR. She was started on four drug antituberculous therapy including Isoniazid, Pyrazinamide, Rifampicin, and Ciprofloxacin, while continuing on CAPD [1].
7. Encapsulating peritoneal sclerosis [EPS] is a rare condition related to vintage of peritoneal dialysis, peritonitis episodes, and exposure to hypertonic glucose solutions. The clinical course is usually described as presymptomatic, inflammatory, and encapsulating ileus. It is associated with high mortality of 50%. Here we present two patients (Fig. 12.7): A 24-year-old male whose contrast CT shows multiloculated collections in the abdomen, peritoneal calcifications, and intra-abdominal hematoma and (Fig. 12.8) a 55-year-old lady who on CAPD for 2 years underwent a deceased donor kidney transplantation. Posttransplant after 8 months she presented with subacute intestinal obstruction. She was treated conservatively. She presented on three occasions with abdominal pain suggestive of intestinal obstruction. CECT showed thickening

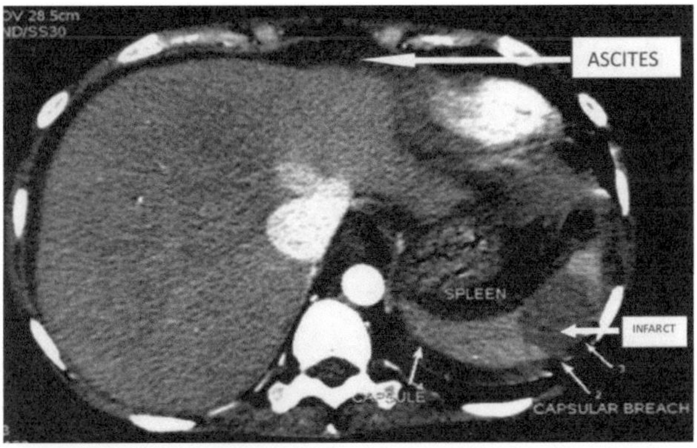

Fig. 12.6 Splenic infarction with capsular breach and hemoperitoneum

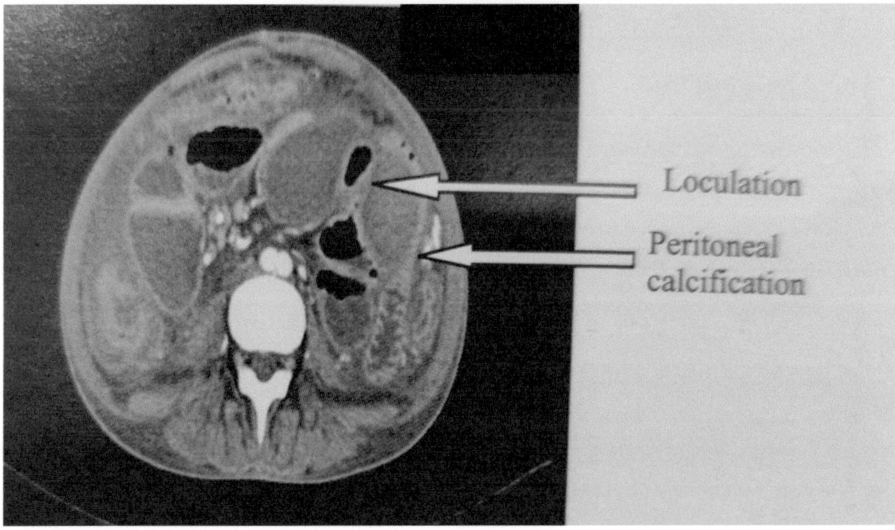

Fig. 12.7 Contrast CT of the abdomen showed multiloculated collections in the abdomen, peritoneal calcification, and intra-abdominal hematoma

of the peritoneal membrane encasing the bowel loops [abdominal cocoon] and gas under the abdominal wall suggestive of intestinal perforation. Laparoscopy showed hard and thickened peritoneum with areas of necrosis encapsulating the intestinal loops. The incidence of EPS is 0.7–3.3%. There is no established treatment modality [2].

8. Pleuroperitoneal communications occur in 1.6–10% of CAPD patients. Patients present with sudden onset of dyspnea, decrease in ultrafiltration, and chest pain. Some may remain asymptomatic or complain of dry cough. Congenital diaphragmatic defects explain the preponderance of right-sided hydrothorax because the left-sided defects are covered by heart and pericardium, hence very little leak. Risk factor for developing hydrothorax includes peritonitis.

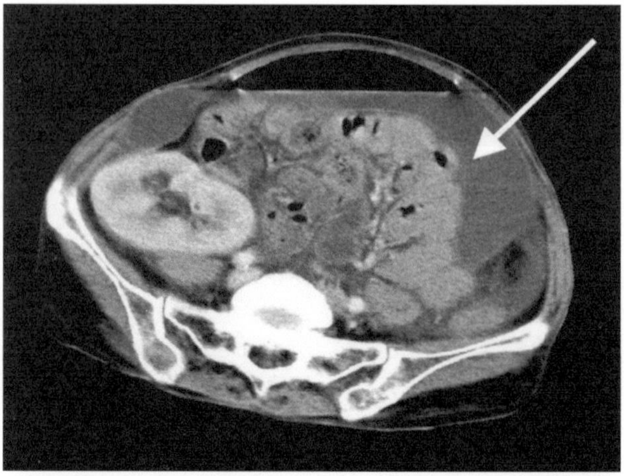

Fig. 12.8 CECT abdomen showing sclerosis of peritoneum[arrow] surrounding the bowel loops and gas beneath the anterior abdominal wall suggestive of pneumoperitoneum

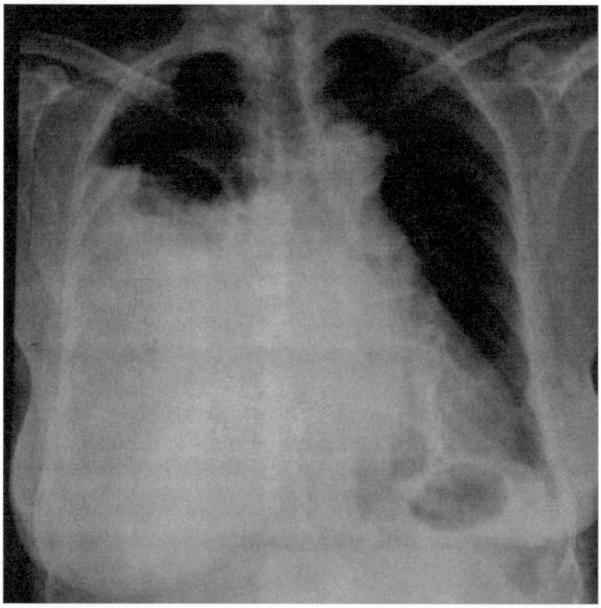

Fig. 12.9 X-ray chest showing right-sided hydrothorax

Here we present the chest radiograph showing massive right-sided hydrothorax (Fig. 12.9). Scintigraphy showed leakage of isotope 99mTC-MAA with instillation of 3 mci of isotope mixed with 300 ml of dialysate and infusion into the peritoneal cavity. Images show abnormal tracer accumulation in the right pleural cavity (Fig. 12.10). As conservative measures failed, a laparoscopic closure of the pleuroperitoneal fistula was done (Fig. 12.11). Nearly 60% of the patients resume maintenance PD after either conservative or interventional treatment. The rest are permanently switched over to hemodialysis [3].

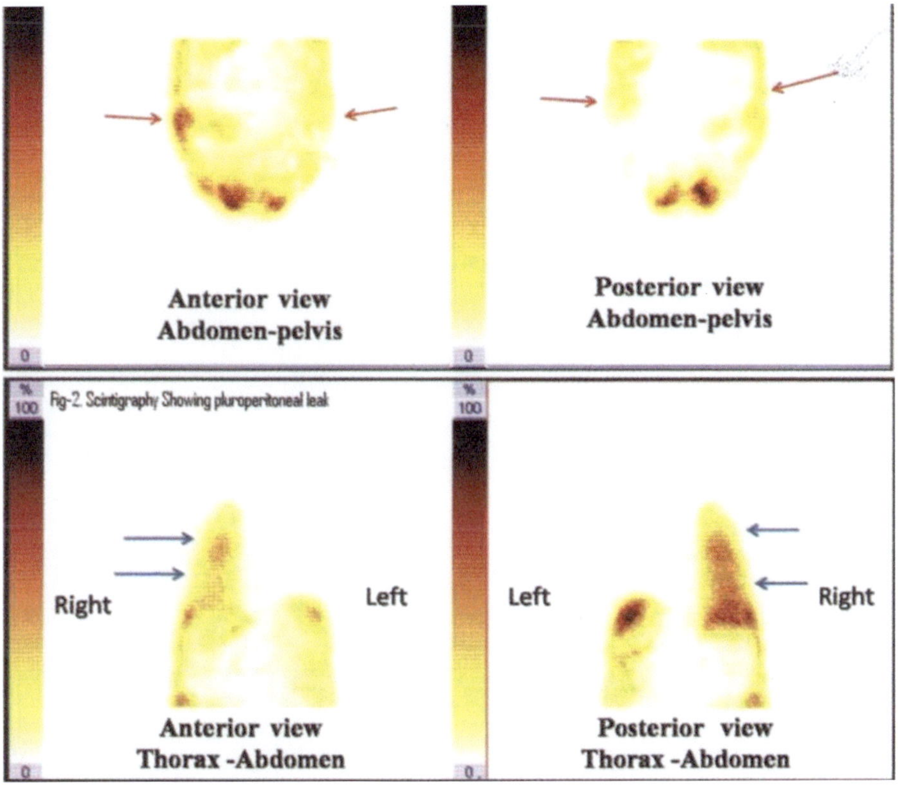

Fig. 12.10 Scintigraphy showing leakage of isotope to right side of chest

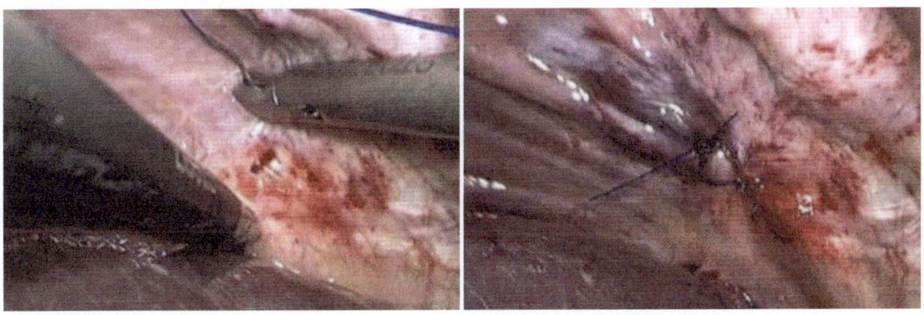

Fig. 12.11 Laparoscopic picture showing pleuroperitoneal fistula and closure

9. Genital edema leading to ultrafiltration failure can occur after an episode of peritonitis. A 10 years old boy on CAPD for 5 years presented with profound genital edema since 2004. Scrotal swelling increased during the process of PD. Figure 12.12 shows bilateral reducible fluctuant scrotal swelling. An abdominal CT with contrast was performed after instilling 1.5% dextrose fluid

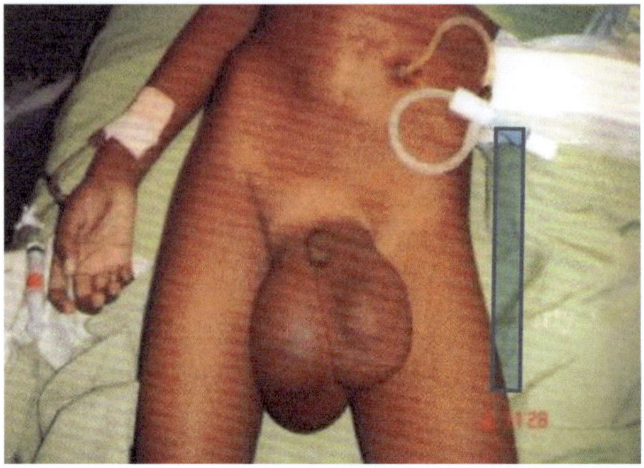

Fig. 12.12 Child with profound genital edema

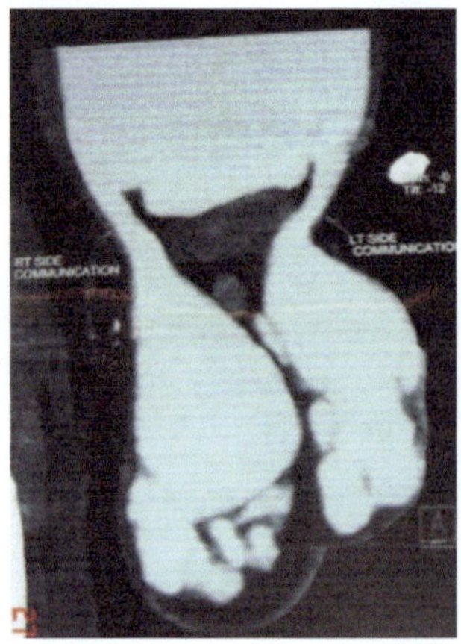

Fig. 12.13 CT scan of abdomen with intraperitoneal contrast instillation showing bilateral patent processus vaginalis with leakage of dialysis fluid

mixed well with 50-60 ml of iohexol into the peritoneal cavity. 64-slice axial CT scan of 5 mm thickness from the diaphragm to upper third of femur concentrating on the scrotal area was done after ambulating the patient for 1 h. The CT scan demonstrated contrast containing dextrose entering the scrotal sac bilaterally establishing the presence of bilateral patent *processus vaginalis* as the cause of genital edema (Fig. 12.13). The child was operated and closure was done. After 4 weeks, he was switched back to CAPD. Genital edema, i.e., edema of scrotum, labia majora, and penis, is seen in 10% of CAPD patients. Genital edema is more common in men compared to women because of the fact that men have increased patency of *processus vaginalis*. The incidence is much higher in children, as high as 25% [4].

10. A 45 years old lady was on PD from October 2013 following a Tenckhoff swan neck catheter implantation. She was doing 2.5% 2 L dextrose 3 times a day. After 3 weeks, she presented with decreased outflow and weight gain of 2 kg. The plain x-ray abdomen showed catheter tip in the pelvis. Few

days later, there was further weight gain of 3.8Kg and lower abdominal wall swelling suggestive of dialysis fluid leak. CT Scan with intraperitoneal contrast showed 4x4mm defect in the left rectus muscle (Fig. 12.14), about 10 cm inferior to the umbilicus in left paramedian location through which fluid was leaking in subcutaneous plane (Fig. 12.15). This leak was treated with low volume exchanges and it sealed by itself without any surgical intervention.

11. A 53 years old hypertensive lady using 2 L dextrose 4 times a day developed an episode of peritonitis in 2003. The culture of the effluent grew *E. coli* and she was treated with intraperitoneal Cefazolin and Ceftazidime in one bag per day. She had no improvement and a repeat dialysis effluent examination showed

Fig. 12.14 CT scan of abdomen showing contrast leak through a defect in left rectus muscle

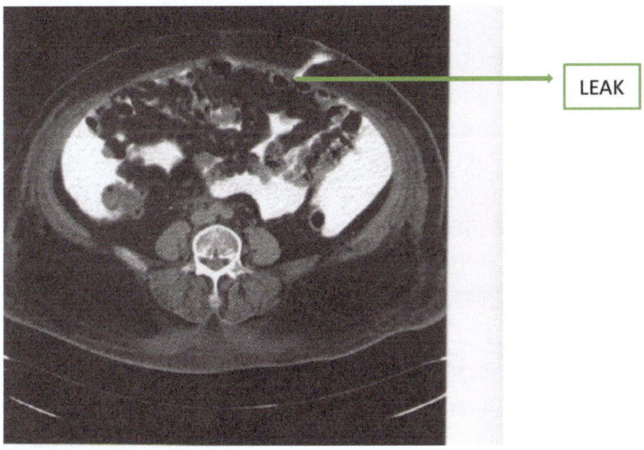

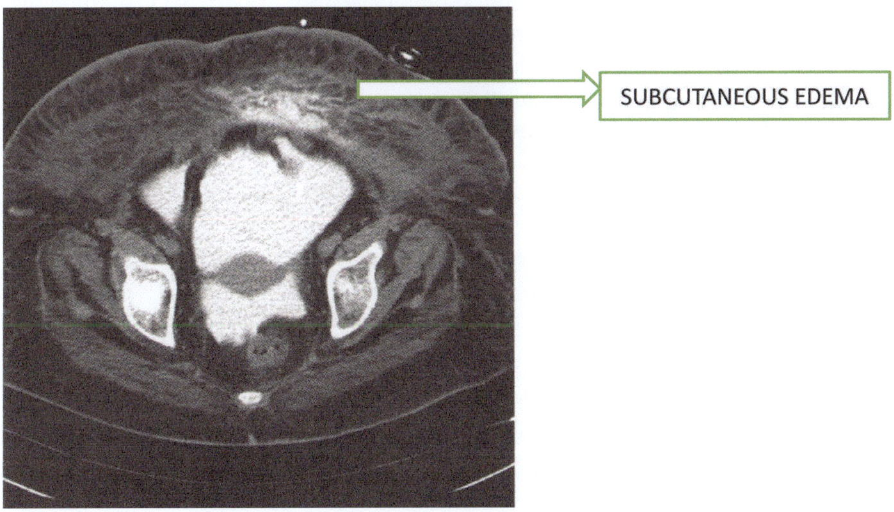

Fig. 12.15 CT scan showing contrast leak and subcutaneous edema

after 18 days *Candida albicans* but no *E. coli*. PD catheter was removed on the third day, and she was transferred to hemodialysis while on intravenous and later oral fluconazole. As the patient wished to go back on PD and there were no symptoms or signs of ongoing peritonitis, a swan neck double cuff Tenckhoff catheter was inserted. A peritoneal biopsy was also taken. The catheter was flushed with dextrose fluid on alternate days, and the effluent did not grow any bacteria or fungus and the drain was clear.

Two liters of dextrose was instilled into the peritoneal cavity 2 weeks after the catheter reimplantation. Only 600 ml of fluid drained out in spite of giving soap and water enema and laxatives. Imaging studies of the abdomen were done. An HRCT scan with contrast instilled into the peritoneal cavity showed tip of the catheter in the left side of pelvis, and the contrast was flowing freely into the peritoneal cavity into a loculation (Fig. 12.16). A repeat HRCT with contrast instilled into 2 liters of fluid showed mesenteric stranding, peritoneal inflammation, and peritoneal omental thickening. PD catheter was removed the next day and patient was switched over to permanent hemodialysis.

CT Scan was a very useful tool in diagnosing adhesions thus avoiding a laparoscopic examination.

12. A 35 years old woman had a swan neck PD catheter implanted after prophylactic antibiotics and bowel preparation. X-ray KUB showed the tip of the catheter in the pelvis. Six hours later, she had hematuria and increased urine output. Ultrasound abdomen showed the tip of the catheter in the urinary bladder (Fig. 12.17). Contrast CT cystography (Fig. 12.18) showed leakage of contrast from the urinary bladder into the dialysis catheter, establishing the diagnosis of bladder perforation during the implantation of the catheter. Laparoscopic placement of a catheter in contrast to bedside blind implantation may avoid this complication of bladder perforation. All patients undergoing either a permanent or temporary catheter implantation should have prior urinary bladder emptying, either through voluntary voiding or by placement of a temporary urinary catheter to ensure an empty bladder. The increased volume of urine while performing PD exchanges should alert the possibility of a bladder penetration. Management consists of removing the PD catheter and leaving an indwelling urinary catheter for a week [5].

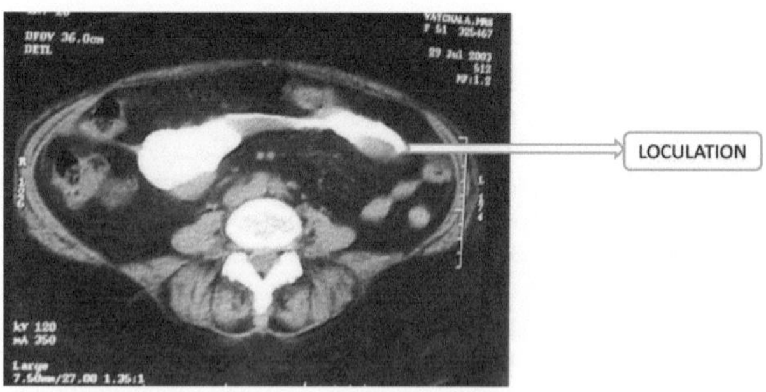

Fig. 12.16 A CT scan with contrast instilled into the peritoneal cavity showed the contrast was flowing into the peritoneal cavity into a loculation

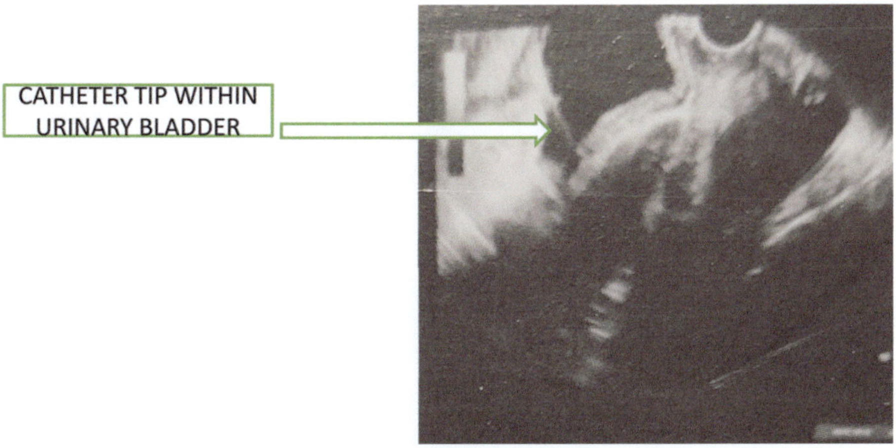

Fig. 12.17 Ultrasound pelvis showing tip of the PD catheter in the urinary bladder

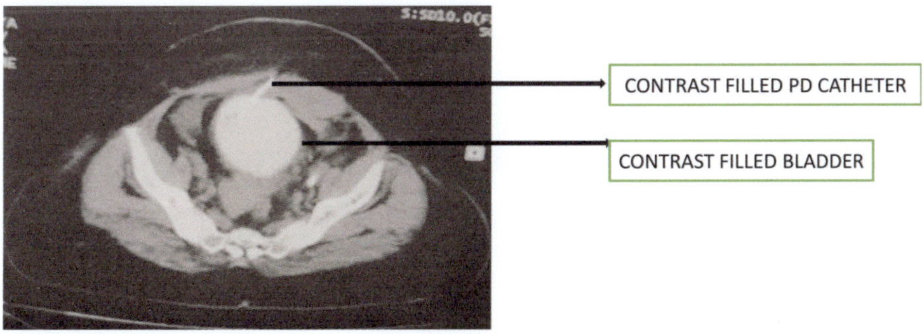

Fig. 12.18 CT cystography showing leakage of contrast from the bladder into the PD catheter

13. A 24-year-old lady on CAPD, using 2 L × 3 exchanges a day, presents with recurrent hemoperitoneum, not been on anticoagulants or antiplatelet drugs. CBC, coagulation bleeding profiles were normal. In the last episode, she had lower abdomen pain with darkish hemoperitoneum. A contrast CT of abdomen was done which showed mild free fluid in pelvis with hyperdense component in dependent portion, suggesting a blood clot/hemoperitoneum (Fig. 12.19). There was a right ovarian cyst which also had dependent hyperdense foci suggestive of blood clot within. The cyst showed wall enhancement (Fig. 12.20), except for a focal area suspicious for wall interruption—suggesting ovarian cyst rupture with secondary hemoperitoneum, which settled with frequent 500 cc flushing with dialysis fluid containing 1000 cc of heparin [6].
14. A 62-year-old male who was on CAPD had an episode of peritonitis and covid-19 infection in 2020. PD catheter was removed and reimplanted and the patient was reinitiated on CAPD. He presented with peritonitis 18 months later which was culture negative. As he developed shock overnight with severe meta-

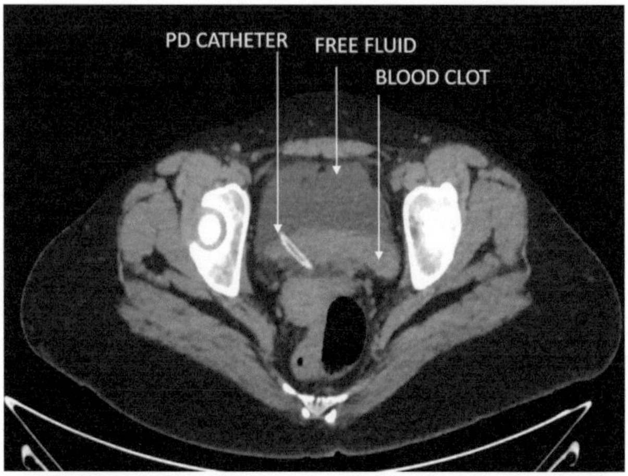

Fig. 12.19 Plain CT of the abdomen shows mild free fluid in pelvis with dependent blood clot

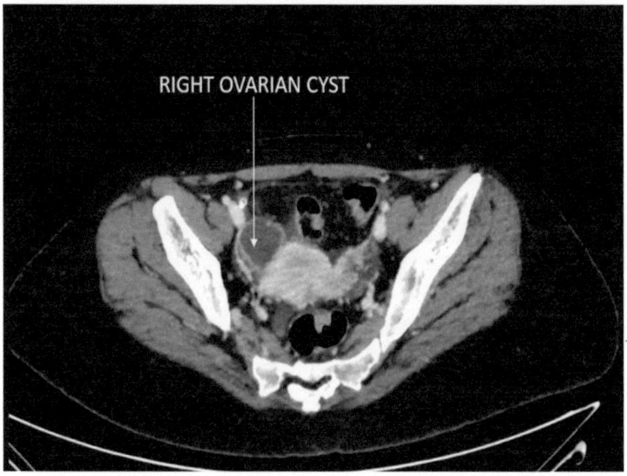

Fig. 12.20 Contrast enhanced CT shows wall enhancement in the right ovarian cyst

bolic acidosis in spite of intraperitoneal Carbapenem and amikacin, a contrast CT of the abdomen was done which showed thrombus in superior mesenteric artery causing small bowel ischemia and ileus (Fig. 12.22). Features of bowel infarction like lack of bowel wall enhancement, pneumatosis intestinalis (Fig. 12.21), mesenteric air, and portal venous gas were present. Emergency laparotomy was done and it revealed extensive ischemia of small bowel. About 105 cm of small intestine was found to be gangrenous, and hence resection anastomosis was done. Coagulation workup was partly done as patient was initiated on heparin and warfarin. The ascites grew *E. coli*. 2D echo of the heart was normal except for left ventricular hypertrophy. He continues on maintenance hemodialysis.

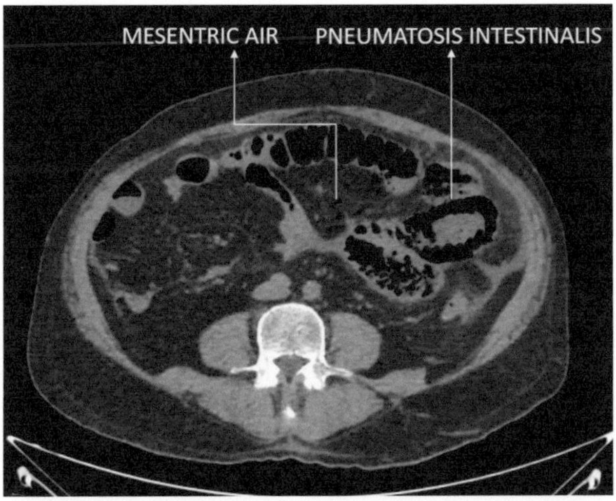

Fig. 12.21 Plain CT shows mesenteric air and intramural air within dilated small bowel loops

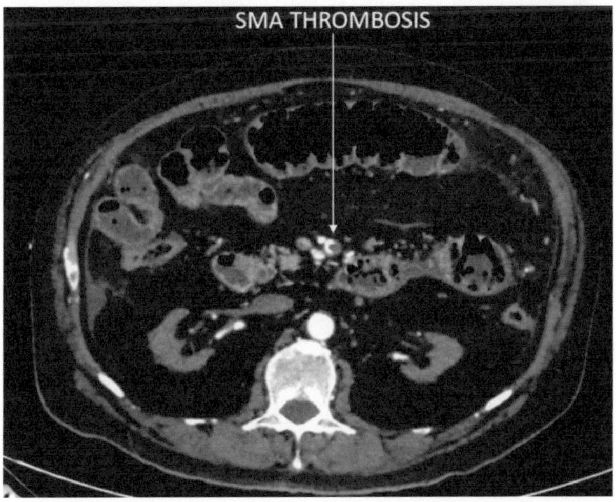

Fig. 12.22 Contrast CT shows SMA thrombosis

12.1 Important Points

Imaging plays an important role in early diagnosis of PD-related complications.

Ultrasound examination of the catheter tunnel is a simple noninvasive technique in evaluating pericatheter leak and infection.

Abdominal and chest radiographs are valuable screening tools in the diagnosis of hydrothorax and in assessment of intraperitoneal catheter position.

CT with and without intraperitoneal contrast is a helpful examination not only to look for pathology of the peritoneum, adhesions, perforations, and leaks but also in prognostication.

[Most of these images are from Indian journal of peritoneal dialysis, Dr. Georgi Abraham being the editor in chief has editorial rights to publish.]

References

1. Blake P, Abraham G, Vas SI, Mathews RE, Oreopoulis DG. Splenic abscess and peritonitis in a CAPD patient. Perit Dial Int. 1989;9:73–4.
2. Moinuddin Z, Summes A, Van Dellen D, Augustine T, Herrick SE. Encapsulating peritoneal sclerosis–a rare but devastating peritoneal disease. Front Physiol. 2015;5:470.
3. Abraham G, Shoker A, Blake P, Orepoulos DG. Massive hydrothorax in patients on peritoneal dialysis. A literature review. Advances in CAPD. Adv Perit Dial. 1988;4:121–5.
4. Abraham G, Blake P, Mathews RE, Izatt S, Oreopoulos DG. Genital swelling as a surgical complication of CAPD. Surg Gynecol Obstet. 1990;170:306–8.
5. Ounissi M, Sfaxi M, Fayala H, Abderrahim E, Abdallah TB, Chebil M, et al. Bladder perforation in a peritoneal dialysis patient. Saudi J Kidney Dis Transpl. 2012;23:552–5.
6. Fraley DS, Johnston JR, Bruns FJ, Adler S, Segel DP. Rupture of ovarian cyst: massive hemoperitoneum in continuous ambulatory peritoneal dialysis patients: diagnosis and treatment. Am J Kidney Dis. 1988 Jul;12(1):69–71. https://doi.org/10.1016/s0272-6386(88)80075-1.

Nutritional Assessment and Management in CAPD Patients with Peritonitis

13

N. Vijayashree, Geroge Kurian, and Kamyar Kalantar-Zadeh

A 51 years old female, nondiabetic, hypertensive diagnosed with end stage kidney disease was on CAPD for 17 years. She presented with *Staphylococcus warneri* peritonitis. She underwent parathyroidectomy for parathyroid hyperplasia. She was treated for *Mycobacterium tuberculous* peritonitis 15 years ago. Her investigations showed Hb- 7.9 g/dl, serum albumin 1.9 g/dl, potassium 2.2 mmol/l, and bicarbonate 28 mmol/l. She was treated with intraperitoneal antibiotic as per ISPD guidelines. Her nutritional assessment showed BMI of 18.9 kg/m^2, and the body composition analysis results showed low skeletal muscle mass (SMM)15.1 kgs (19.3–23.5kgs), soft lean mass (SLM) 28.8 kgs (33.4–40.8 kgs), fat free mass (FFM) 31.2 kgs (35.4–43.3kgs), and low body cell mass (BCM) of 18.8 kgs (23.1–28.3kgs). Subjective global assessment (SGA) was used to analyze the nutritional status which showed severe malnutrition due to loss of appetite, restriction of physical functional capacity, diarrhea, and increased metabolic demand. The dietary intake was 772 kcal and 22gms of protein per day, and current nutritional status diagnosed urgent nutritional support as the ongoing malnutrition worsened by protracted peritonitis. A nutritional plan was prescribed to have 1800 kcals at 35 kcals/kg/day and 70gms of protein at 1.5gm/kg of ideal body weight per day. Oral nutrition support was initiated to improve the nutrient intake. There was an increase in energy and protein intake to 1200 kcals and 30 gms, which was insufficient to meet the requirement. She had diarrhea and abdominal distention, oral feeds were unable

N. Vijayashree (✉) · G. Kurian · K. Kalantar-Zadeh
MGM Healthcare, Chennai, Tamil Nadu, India

Matha Amritha Hospital, Kochi, India

Irvine School of Medicine, Irvine, CA, USA
e-mail: kkz@hs.uci.edu

G. Abraham et al. (eds.), *Diagnosis and Management of Complications of Peritoneal Dialysis related Peritonitis*,
https://doi.org/10.1007/978-981-99-2275-8_13

to meet the recommended dietary allowances (RDA), and she was given an additional nutrition support through intradialytic parenteral nutrition (IDPN—986 ml per dialysis) weekly twice for 4 weeks during her time on intermittent hemodialysis. This provided an addition of 1100 kcals and 50gms protein. The total intake of the patient was 2000 kcals and 80 gms of protein, which was meeting the RDA along with micronutrient supplementation. Patient's nutritional status improved and was able to meet recommended calories and protein with the help of oral nutrition supplement. Follow-up body composition analysis showed gradual improvement in skeletal muscle mass (SMM) to 16 kgs, soft lean mass (SLM) 29.7 kgs, and fat free mass (FFM) 32.1 kgs. Similarly, as shown in Fig. 13.1, the albumin levels were increased from 1.9gd/l to 3.4 g/dl during 2 months follow-up. Currently, patient is weighing 52 kgs leading a quality life. The PD regimen was modified to 2 L × 1 bag of icodextrin and 2 × 2L liters bag of (7.5%) dianeal. Patient has no further episode of peritonitis.

This longest living home PD patient in India with previous peritoneal dialysis-related *Mycobacterium tuberculous* peritonitis with many nutritional issues has regained her adequate nutritional status through intense nutrition therapy, frequent diet counseling by a trained renal nutritionist, adequate dialysis prescription, family support, and positive attitude of the patient (Fig. 13.2).

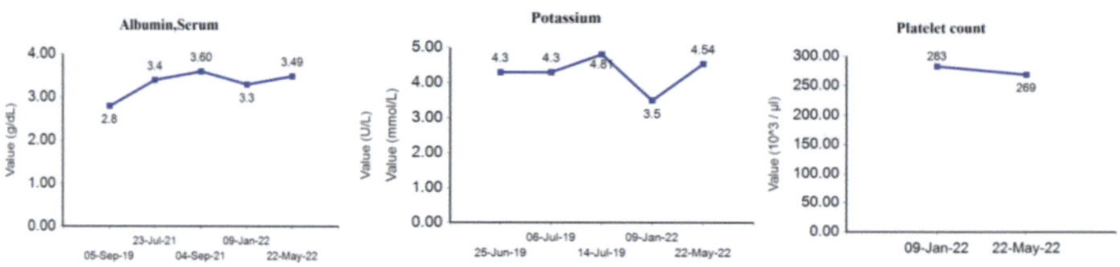

Fig. 13.1 Analysis of biochemical parameters

Fig. 13.2 Wasted subcutaneous tissue and prominent distal cuff

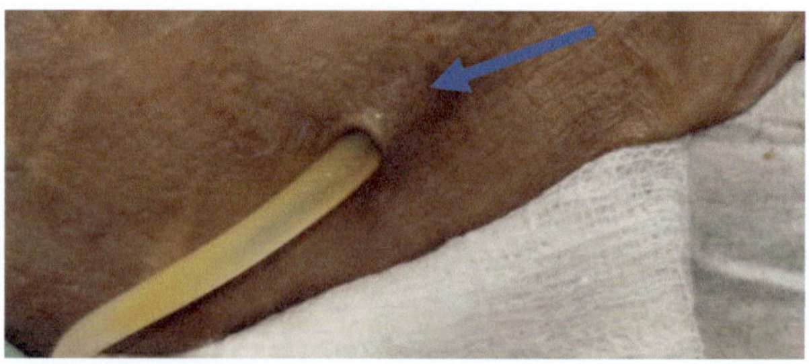

A 42 years old lady on CAPD for 5 years had *E. coli* peritonitis, which was successfully treated. Her serum albumin was 2.9 g/dl. Her prior albumin level was 3.8 g/dl. She required intense nutritional support, and picture 2 shows loss of subcutaneous fat and prominence of distal cuff suggesting protein energy malnutrition.

13.1 Nutritional Assessment and Care

The nutritional status of the patients has a greater impact on the management of peritonitis in CAPD patients, and the ongoing malnutrition can worsen the peritonitis due to hypokalemia, hypoalbuminemia, hypophosphatemia, and lack of immune-related nutrition support. Malnutrition can also be worsened by the prolonged in tunnel infection due to the inflammation and antibiotic use in peritonitis. Protein energy malnutrition (PEW) is significant in case of prolonged peritonitis. Early nutritional assessment and treatment of nutritional problems in CAPD may lead to overall better outcome. Many guidelines exist regarding assessment of nutrition and management of nutrition in patients with CKD and on dialysis as shown in Fig. 13.3. There is no single measurement or assessment that can be used to determine the presence of malnutrition; hence a panel of anthropometric measurements and biochemical parameters are recommended [1].

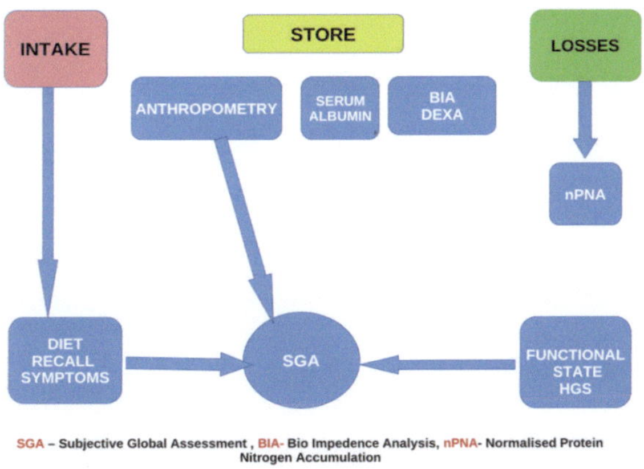

Fig. 13.3 Nutritional assessment and management

13.2 Subjective Global Assessment (SGA)

Subjective global assessment (SGA) is a tool that uses five components of a medical history (weight change, dietary intake, gastrointestinal symptoms, physical functional capacity, and metabolic demand) and three components of a brief physical examination (signs of fat and muscle wasting, nutrition-associated alternations in fluid balance) to assess nutritional status.

The SGA has been found to be a valid and reliable tool for assessing PEW. A single SGA assessment has shown presence of malnutrition and was found to be associated with morbidity, hospitalization, and mortality in several clinical studies. Therefore, since 2000 the National Kidney Foundation Kidney Disease/Dialysis Outcomes and Quality Initiative (K/DOQI) has recommended the use of the SGA for assessing the nutritional status of dialysis patients.

13.3 Malnutrition Inflammation Score (MIS)

MIS is the modified version of SGA for dialysis patients. The MIS is an inexpensive and easy tool to assess score of 0 to 30 to diagnose protein—energy wasting (PEW) and inflammation as shown in Table 13.1. The seven components of the SGA and additional BMI, serum albumin, and TIBC are valid tools. The results are obtained from the simple sum of each of the items, finally expressing them into the following categories [2]:

Table 13.1 MIS Interpretation [3]

Classification	MIS score
Normally nourished	0–2
Mild malnutrition	3–5
Moderate malnutrition	6–8
Severe malnutrition	Above

13.4 Anthropometric Measurements

Anthropometrics are objective measurements that help to determine the amount of muscle mass and body fat. It is inexpensive, non-invasive, and easy to perform. Measurements may include height, weight, BMI, skinfold thickness, body composition measures (BCM), fat folds, and hip and waist circumferences. It has to be repeated periodically for longitudinal assessment as the changes are not obvious for 3–4 weeks

13.5 Body Mass Index

The BMI is a convenient rule of thumb used to broadly categorize a person as *underweight*, *normal weight*, *overweight*, or *obese*. Major adult BMI classifications are (Table 13.2) underweight (under 18.5 kg/m2), normal (18.5 to 24.9 kg/m2), for South Asians (18.5–22.9 kg/m^2), overweight (25 to 29.9 kg/m2), and obese (30 kg/m2 or more). BMI has limitations in interpretation especially when applied to individuals with abdominal obesity, short stature, high muscle mass, and sarcopenia.

Weight Loss Percentage
Unintentional weight loss is considered as a risk for malnutrition (Table 13.3).

Table 13.2 WHO BMI classification, 2020 [3]

BMI = Weight in kg/height in m^2	
Classification	BMI Asian
Underweight	<18.50
Severe thinness	<16.00
Moderate thinness	16.00–16.99
Mild thinness	17.00–18.49
Normal range	18.50–22.99
Overweight	≥23.00
Pre-obese	23.00–27.99
Obese	≥27.00
Obese class I	27.00–30.99
Obese class II	30.00–34.99
Obese class III	≥34.00

Table 13.3 Weight loss percentage

Weight loss % = (Usual body weight—current body weight)/(usual body weight) × 100		
Time	Significant weight loss (%)	Severe weight loss (%)
1 week	1–2%	>2%
1 month	5%	>5%
3 months	7.5%	>7.5%
6 months	10%	>10%

13.6 Skinfold Thickness

Skinfold thickness (SFT) measurement (Fig. 13.4) is a simple, non-invasive method of body fat estimation at all ages including the new-born period. It measures the thickness of subcutaneous fat at various sites of the body. It is compared with percentile standards from multiple body sites which are collected over time; triceps, biceps, subscapular, and suprailiac using calipers are most commonly used (Fig. 13.5).

The following are the nine anatomical sites that are most commonly used in the assessment of fat by skinfold thickness measures:

(a) *Chest or pectoral skinfold:* For men, get a diagonal fold halfway between the armpit and the nipple. For women, a diagonal fold 1/3 of the way from the arm pit to the nipple
(b) *Mid-axillary:* A vertical fold on the mid-axillary line which runs directly down from the center of the armpit
(c) *Suprailiac or flank:* A diagonal fold just above the front forward protrusion of the hip bone
(d) *Abdominal:* A horizontal fold about 3 cm to the side of the midpoint of the umbilicus and 1 cm below umbilicus

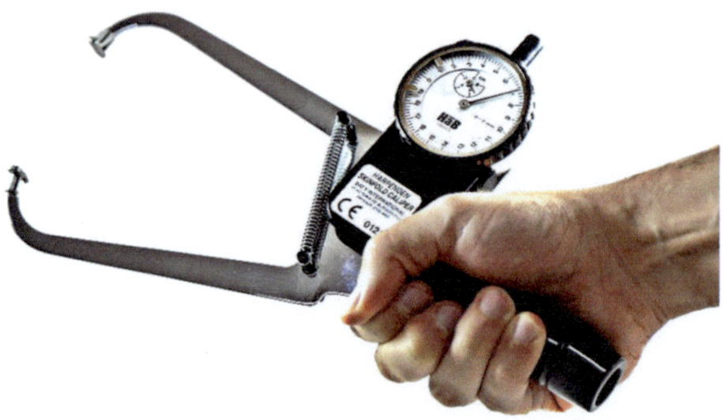

Fig. 13.4 Harpenden caliper

(e) *Quadriceps or mid-thigh:* A vertical fold midway between the knee and top of the thigh
(f) *Triceps:* A vertical fold midway between the acromion process and the olecranon process at the elbow
(g) *Biceps:* A vertical pinch mid-biceps at the same level the triceps skinfold was taken
(h) *Subscapular:* A diagonal fold just below the inferior angle of the scapula
(i) *Medial Calf:* The foot is placed flat on an elevated surface with the knee flexed at a 90° angle. A vertical fold taken at the widest point of the calf at the medial or inner aspect of the calf [4]

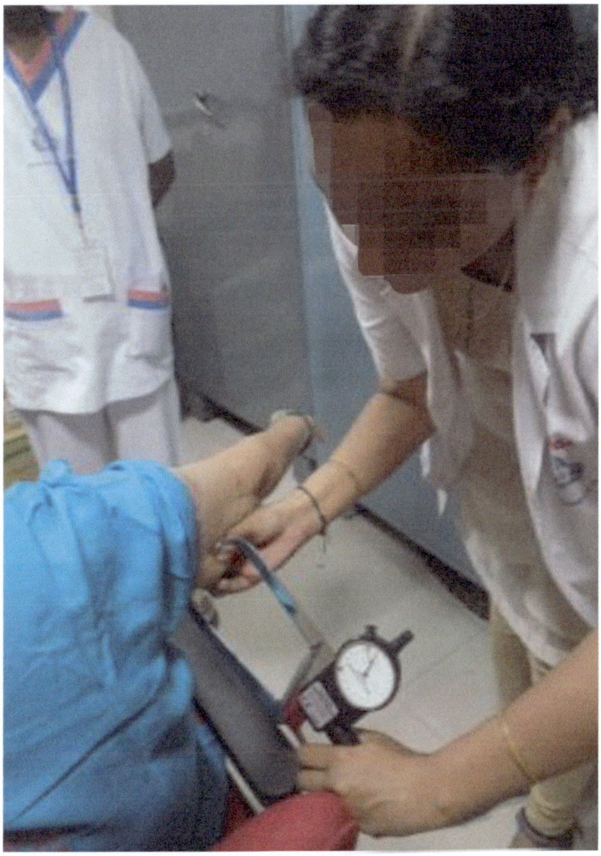

Fig. 13.5 Triceps skinfold thickness

Table 13.4 Mid-arm muscle circumference cut-off

MAMC = (MAC) − (TSF × 3.14)	
Level of under nutrition	MAMC (mm)
Moderate	<185 mm
Severe	<160 mm

FANTA (Food and Nutrition Technical Assistance) Global MAUC cut-offs for adult: A technical consultation, 2018

13.7 Mid-arm Muscle Circumference

Mid-arm muscle circumference estimates somatic protein stores (skeletal muscle mass) and body fat stores. Mid-arm muscle circumference (MAMC): determined from the mid-arm circumference (MAC) and triceps skinfold (TSF). Mid-arm muscle mass provides a good indication of lean body mass, used in the estimation of upper arm fat area. The cutoff is given in Table 13.4 [5].

13.8 Hand Grip Strength (HGS)

Handgrip strength is an easily performed simple bedside test that has been shown to correlate with lean body mass in patients with CAPD (Fig. 13.6). It reflects body lean muscle mass and predicts survival. Studies in general population groups reported a similar association between a low HGS and poor nutritional status. There is also recent evidence that HGS may be a powerful predictor of disability, morbidity, and mortality [4].

Hand grip strength, also correlates with elbow flexion strength, knee extension strength, and trunk extension strength and thus gives an approximation of muscle mass. The patients were instructed to apply as much hand grip pressure as possible by using the hand without AV fistula. The measurements were repeated three times and the average score was recorded in kilograms [4].

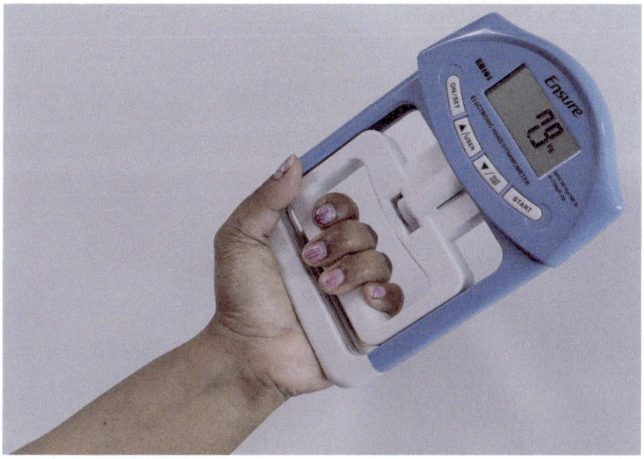

Fig. 13.6 Handgrip dynamometer

13.9 Body Composition Measures (BCM)

Human body is composed of water, protein, mineral, and body fat, the sum of which becomes body weight. BCM is considered as the most reliable tool that helps to find out the body fat percentage, lean body mass, skeletal muscle mass, mineral mass, total body water, intracellular water (ICW), extracellular water (ECW), body cell mass, arm muscle circumference, visceral fat area, and basal metabolic rate. By passing electrical currents at the end of limbs and by measuring the voltage, the impedance of each segment can be obtained (Figs. 13.7, 13.8, and 13.9).

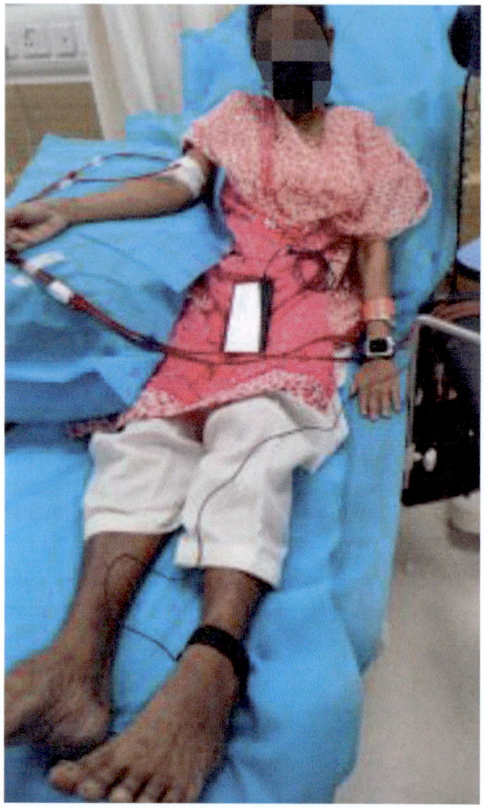

Fig. 13.7 Measuring body composition

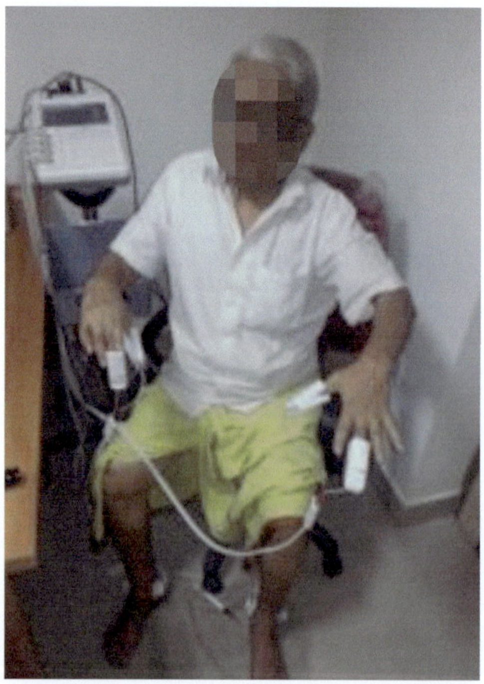

Fig. 13.8 Measuring body composition

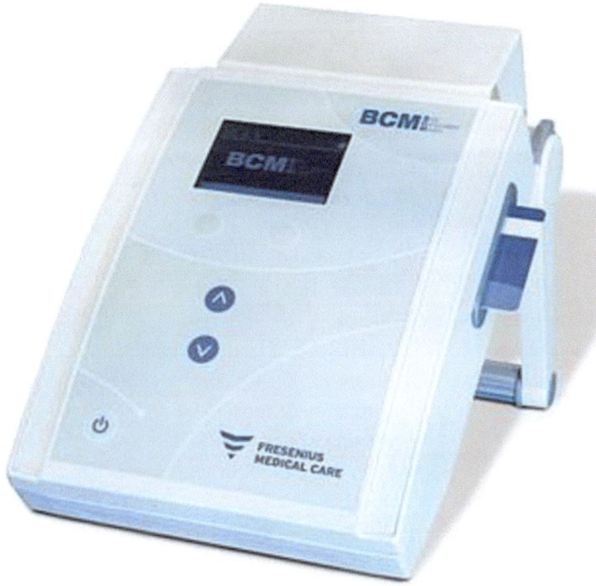

Fig. 13.9 Body composition analyzer

13.10 Dual Energy X-Ray Absorptiometry (DEXA)

DEXA scan is the most reliable, non-invasive method to assess the three main components of body composition—fat mass—fat-free mass—bone mineral mass and density. It is less influenced by hydration and has superior precision and accuracy compared to anthropometry.

13.11 Biochemical Parameters

Serum albumin and pre-albumin have by far been the most commonly used marker of nutritional status in patients on PD with peritonitis. Following are the laboratory tests which help to evaluate the nutritional status:

Visceral proteins—Albumin, pre-albumin, transferrin, and amino acids
Lipids—Cholesterol, triglycerides
Somatic protein and nitrogen—BUN and creatinine
Growth factor IGF and leptin
Peripheral CBC, lymphocytes
C- reactive protein

Table 13.5 Clinical observation and nutrient deficiencies

Area/system	Symptom or sign	Deficiency
General	Wasting	Energy
Skin	Rash	Vitamins, zinc, EFAs
	Rash (sun exposure)	Niacin
Hair	Thinning or loss	Protein
	Premature whitening	Selenium
Nails	Spooning	Iron
Eyes	Impaired night vision	Vitamin A
Mouth	Cheilosis and glossitis	Riboflavin, niacin, B6, iron
Extremities	Edema	Protein
Neurologic	Psychological issues	B12 deficiencies
	Tetany	Ca+, mg+
	Limitation of movements	Protein, vitamin D
MSK	Wasting of muscle	Protein
	Bone deformities & tenderness	Vitamin D, calcium
GI	Diarrhea	Protein, niacin, folate, B12
	Diarrhea and dysgeusia	Zinc
	Dysphagia/odynophagia	Iron
Endocrine	Thyromegaly	Iodine

EFA Essential fatty acids, *MSK* musculoskeletal, *GI* gastrointestinal

13.12 Clinical Observation

A clinical assessment by inspecting head to toe by treating nephrologist and renal nutritionist can unmask many deficiencies. It identifies the physical signs of malnutrition (e.g., temporal wasting, facial muscle atrophy) and micronutrient deficiencies. Signs do not appear unless severe deficiencies exist. Most signs/symptoms indicate two or more deficiencies (Table 13.5).

13.13 Dietary Assessment

Evaluating the energy and protein intake and source of protein helps the dietician to alter and plan a diet for CKD patients. Diet history can be obtained by using the following:

- *24 h dietary recall method*
- *Food frequency and various food logs*
- *Food diary*

Protein Equivalent of Total Nitrogen Appearance (PNA) or Protein Catabolic Rate (PCR)

PCR is a good indirect index for dietary protein intake, expressed as gm/day. It is calculated by

$$\text{Protein catabolic rate}\left(\text{g / day}\right)=\left[\left(\mathbf{24-h\,urine\ urea\ nitrogen+4}\right)^{*}\mathbf{6.25}\right]$$

based on 6.25 g protein yielding 1 g nitrogen.

PNA or PCR is a valid and clinically useful measure of net protein degradation dietary protein and dietary energy intake in dialysis patients.

13.14 Nutrition Management in Peritonitis

Twenty-four hours protein loss and amino acid loss in CAPD is 5–15gm and 2–4gm/day, respectively. Peritonitis is a major infective complication in which increased peritoneal protein and amino acid loss increased to manyfold, if protracted leads to major morbidity and sometimes mortality. This calls for meticulous nutritional intervention, and when the functioning gut is at compromise, total parenteral nutrition as in our patient should be advocated. Appetite enhancing agents can be added for improving nutritional status. The nutritional requirement for CAPD patient with peritonitis is given in Table 13.7.

13.15 Energy Requirement

Due to increased catabolism, patients should be provided adequate non-protein calories. Complex carbohydrate and essential fatty acids are considered as the best source of energy. In people with peritonitis, 30–35 kcals per kg body dry weight is recommended. Patients should be monitored once a week to assess for energy, protein, and micronutrient intake and fluid status due to ultrafiltration problems along with BCM for fluid status.

13.16 Proteins

Patients on CAPD already have high protein requirements due to loss of protein through the dialysis process. In PD peritonitis, protein loss can increase up to 70% due to hypercatabolism, leading to weight loss, as a result of breakdown of body's muscle stores. The protein requirement during peritonitis is 1.2–1.5gm/kg body weight. Fifty percentage of the protein should be of high biological value protein (HBV). This can be achieved by two ways:

- Home-/kitchen-made protein foods
- Oral nutrition supplements

Table 13.6 Protein content and biological value of foods

Animal sources	Protein content/100gm	Biological value %	Plant source	Protein content/100gm	Biological value %
Whole egg	10 g	100	Whey protein isolate	87 g	100
White egg	12 g	98	Soya	37.8 g	96
Chicken	18 g	79	Pulses	5 g	49
Lean meat	24 g	74	Nuts	20 g	45
Fish	18 g	83	Wheat	13 g	64
Cow's milk and milk products	3.4 g	91	Rice	2.7 g	83
			Millets	6 g	52
			Sprouts	5 g	80

13.17 Protein Food Sources

There are two types of protein in the foods we eat: animal protein and vegetable (plant) protein. Animal proteins are easier for your body to use, but most people need both types of protein in their diet. Here are some examples of foods high in protein with their biological value in Table 13.6 [6].

HBV of the foods can be increased by combining different foods, because the different components favor each other:

- 85% rice and 15% yeast: 118 HBV score
- 55% soy and 45% rice: 111 HBV score
- 55% potatoes and 45% soy: 103 HBV score
- 52% beans and 48% corn: 101 HBV score.

13.18 Effect of Germination on Protein Digestibility and Availability

Germination is a simple method which also improves the biological value of proteins. It is commonly practiced in Indian kitchen. Digestibility of protein, crucial in determining the protein quality of food, was increased by 14–18% after germination of green gram, cowpea, lentil, and chickpeas.

Pulses are consumed worldwide and are desired for their high protein quality and quantity. They represent an affordable alternative to animal protein by complementing cereal proteins, thus providing a balanced amino acid profile in vegetarian diets. However, the nutritional benefits of pulse proteins may be limited by antinutrients and protease inhibitors which form complexes with proteins and proteolytic enzymes, reducing the bioavailability and digestibility of dietary protein. Germination can reduce the detrimental effect of these antinutritional factors and allow the full dietary benefits of cereal and pulse proteins to be realized. The availability of crude protein and essential amino acids increase substantially during germination by up to 21% and 52–76% of total protein and essential amino acids, respectively.

13.19 Nutritional Supplements

In order to meet high protein and energy requirements, it is likely that peritonitis patients will require nutritional supplements. Several factors contribute to lower dietary intake among peritonitis patients, including anorexia, inadequate dialysis, volume overload, gastrointestinal disease, and comorbid illness. Administration of oral nutritional supplements would have beneficial effects on the nutritional status among these patients.

The implementation of dietary interventions can be challenging to the medical care team and patients. Supplementary HBV protein induces a significant improvement in energy and protein intake, serum albumin concentration, muscle strength, and quality of life. Therefore, oral-specific renal nutritional supplementation is designed to increase energy, protein, and fiber intake and decrease the intake of sodium, potassium, and phosphorus to improve outcomes.

13.20 Potassium

Potassium, a cation predominantly intracellular (150 mmol/l), is needed to keep the nerves, muscles, and heart function. Low or high potassium can cause cardiac arrythmias and cardiac arrest. CAPD patients usually maintain their serum potassium within normal range of 3.5–5 mmol/l. However, during severe peritonitis due to inadequate intake, indigestion and PD losses may lead to hypokalemia and attendant complications. The potassium requirement of a patient is 40–70 mmol/day. Hyperkalemia (potassium >5 mmol/l) may develop in the anuric patients consuming high potassium containing food stuffs.

13.21 Phosphate

Too much phosphorus in the blood may make the bones weak and likely to break and may make the skin itchy. Peritoneal dialysis may not remove enough phosphorus, so it needs to limit foods which are high in phosphorus, and ingestion of phosphate binder is necessary to control the phosphorus in the blood. Common phosphate binders include sevelamer carbonate, calcium acetate, lanthanum carbonate, and calcium carbonate. These bind phosphorus in the diet thereby reducing the absorption. The dietary phosphorus intake should be restricted to 800–1000 mg/day to ensure phosphorus homeostasis. A low phosphorus protein ratio diet should be advised.

The lowest amount of phosphorus in proportion to the quantity and quality of protein comes from animal flesh proteins (average, 11 mg of phosphorus per 1gm of protein), whereas eggs, dairy products, legume, and lentils have higher phosphorus-protein ratios (average 20 mg of phosphorus per 1gm of protein).

Food industries often add phosphorus to processed and packaged foods, such as baked and processed foods. These food items should be limited or avoided by the CKD patients. Poultry, fish, nuts, peanut butter, dried beans, cola, tea, and dairy products are high in phosphorus. In grossly malnourished peritonitis patients, hypophosphatemia ($P < 2.2$ mg/dl) may occur and assessment should be done to unmask this (Table 13.7) [7].

Table 13.7 Recommended nutrient intake of patients on peritoneal dialysis

Nutrient	Recommendation PD	Recommendation Peritonitis
Protein	1.2–1.3 g/kg/d	1.2–1.5 g/kg/d
Calories	25–35 kcl/kg/d	30–35 kcl/kg/d
Fat (% of total energy)	30–40	30–40
Fiber intake	20–25 g/d	20–25 g/d
Sodium	2 g/d	2 g/d
Potassium	40–70 mEq	40–70 mEq
Calcium	1000 mg/d	1000 mg/d
Magnesium	200–300 mg/d	200–300 mg/d
Phosphorus	800–1000 mg/d	800–1000 mg/d
Zinc	15 mg/d	15 mg/d
Thiamine	1.5 mg/d	1.5 mg/d
Riboflavin	1.8 mg/d	1.8 mg/d
Pantothenic acid	5.0 mg/d	5.0 mg/d
Niacin	20 mg/d	20 mg/d
Pyridoxine	10 mg/d	10 mg/d
Vitamin B12	3 μg/d	3 μg/d
Vitamin C	60 mg/d	60 mg/d
Folic acid	1 mg/d	1 mg/d
Vitamin A E K	No addition	No addition
Vitamin D	Calcitriol as required	Calcitriol as required

Source: Abraham Georgi et al, Management of Malnutrition in CKD in South Asia, 2018

13.22 Intradialytic Parenteral Nutrition (IDPN)

IDPN is used as a nutritional treatment in the catabolic, dialyzed patients. It is safe and efficient when carefully used over a 6-month period in trying to attenuate existing or worsening malnutrition in these patients. It should be commenced at an early stage in these patients, after attempts at oral nutritional support have been deemed inadequate. In acutely ill patients with CKD on dialysis, the goal of parenteral nutrition (PN) is to reduce protein catabolism and nutritional depletion-associated morbidity and mortality. In undernourished CAPD patients while switching over to maintenance hemodialysis, initiation of IDPN improves the quality of life by ameliorating PEW-related complications, hospitalization, and mortality.

13.23 Nutritional Recommendations for Pediatric Patients Treated with Peritoneal Dialysis

Children have unique nutritional demands. Inadequate nutritional status in children younger than 5 years of age results in poor growth leading to development of health disparities. What is more important is nutrition plays a vital role in the development of the brain during the postnatal and preschool periods, as neurons undergo rapid development and synaptic pruning during the first 5 years of life. Children who suffer from CKD have impaired nutritional status directly resulting in sub-optimal growth. This may be attributed to growth hormone and insulin-like growth factor I axis dysregulation, metabolic acidosis, anemia, nutritional deficiencies, renal osteodystrophy, and inflammation. The nutritional requirements of the pediatric CAPD patients are given in Table 13.8 [8, 9].

Table 13.8 Recommended Energy and Protein Intake of Children

Age	Energy (kcal/kg/day)	Protein (g/kg/day)
Peritoneal dialysis (CCPD/CAPD) Infants Preterm	120–180	3.0–4.0
0–0.5 year	115–150	2.1–3.0
0.5–1.0 years	95–150	2.0–3.0
1.0–2.0 years	95–120	2.0–3.0
Children/ adolescents 2.0 years of puberty	Minimum of EAR (estimated average requirement)	2.5
Pubertal	According to height age	2.0
Post-pubertal	According to height age	1.5

Source: Abraham Georgi et al, Management of Malnutrition in CKD in South Asia, 2018 [7]

Key Points

- Malnutrition is common in home peritoneal dialysis patients especially during peritonitis.
- Presence of peritonitis worsens the state of malnutrition leading to increased morbidity and mortality.
- A trained renal nutritionist/dietitian should assess the nutritional status frequently using anthropometric, clinical, biochemical, and dietary assessment.
- As vegetarian diet may not provide enough high biological value proteins (HBVP), which should be 50% of the total protein intake, every effort should be put in to overcome this problem.
- Oral nutritional supplement which has both macro- and micronutrients may be given to overcome the deficiencies.
- Dyselectrolytemia such as hypokalemia and hypo- and hyperphosphatemia should be addressed.
- Follow-up nutritional assessment with 3 days of dietary recall, anthropometric, and biochemical parameters is important for good quality of life in patients with peritonitis.

References

1. Kiebalo T, Holotka J, Habura I, Pawlaczyk K. Nutritional status in peritoneal dialysis: nutritional guidelines, adequacy and the Management of Malnutrition. Poznan, Poland: Department of Nephrology, Transplantology and Internal Medicine, Poznan University of Medical Sciences; 2020. p. 60–355.
2. Kalantar-Zadeh K, et al. Malnutrition-inflammation complex syndrome in dialysis patients: causes and consequences. Am J Kidney Dis. 2003;42(5):864–81.
3. WHO BMI classification, 2020.
4. Tian M, Zha Y, Li Q, Yuan J. Handgrip strength and mortality in maintenance Haemodialysis patients. Guiyang, China: Department of Nephrology, Guizhou Provincial People's Hospital; 2019.
5. FANTA (Food and Nutrition Technical Assistance) Global MAUC cutoffs for adult: a technical consultation, 2018.
6. Shiksha A, et al. Protein quality in perspective: a review of protein quality metrics and their applications. Nutrients. 2022;14(5):947.
7. Abraham Georgi et al, Management of Malnutrition in CKD in South Asia, 2018.
8. KDOQI Work Group. KDOQI Clinical practice guideline for nutrition in children with CKD. Am J Kidney Dis. 2008;53(3):S1–S124.
9. KDOQI clinical practice guidelines for nutrition in Chronic Kidney disease, 2020.

Special Challenges with Peritonitis in Children

14

Nivedita Kamath and Arpana Iyengar

Case Vignettes

1. A 12-year-old boy with neurogenic bladder and kidney failure on peritoneal dialysis (PD) was admitted with cloudy effluent. The fluid analysis showed 1970 cells with 95% neutrophils. The culture of the fluid, however, did not isolate any organism. He was treated with intraperitoneal antibiotics (Cefepime). The fluid analysis after 5 days of therapy showed a total count of 5 cells and the same antibiotic therapy was continued. He also received fluconazole as prophylaxis against fungal infection. Five days later, he came with increasing abdominal pain and cloudy effluent. The fluid analysis showed 2040 cells and 92% neutrophils. He was started on Ceftazidime and Amikacin. The culture did not isolate any bacterial or fungal organisms. He received antibiotic therapy for 3 weeks. The cell count on day 5 of therapy had reduced to 25 cells. He was diagnosed to have relapsing peritonitis.
2. A 9-year-old girl with bilateral hypodysplastic kidneys with kidney failure has been on PD for the last 3 years. She had two episodes of peritonitis in the last 6 months. The first episode was a culture-negative peritonitis that was treated with intraperitoneal antibiotics and resolved with treatment. About 2 months later, she had another episode of peritonitis. Acinetobacter was isolated and she received weeks of therapy with Meropenem. After 5 days of therapy, the fluid analysis showed 500 cells with 80% neutrophils. The culture test was repeated and it isolated Candida parapsilosis. The PD catheter was removed and she was switched to hemodialysis. She received 3 weeks of Amphotericin B therapy. This is an example of a child with fungal peritonitis.

N. Kamath (✉) · A. Iyengar
Department of Pediatric Nephrology, St John's Medical College Hospital, Bangalore, Karnataka, India

G. Abraham et al. (eds.), *Diagnosis and Management of Complications of Peritoneal Dialysis related Peritonitis*,
https://doi.org/10.1007/978-981-99-2275-8_14

14.1 Introduction

Peritoneal dialysis (PD) remains the preferred modality of dialysis in children with kidney failure. Advances in PD connectology, quality improvement measures like PD care bundles have significantly reduced the risk of complications. However, peritonitis continues to be the most important complication of PD that contributes to morbidity and technique failure [1, 2].

Multiple episodes of peritonitis are associated with reduced function of the peritoneal membrane and increased risk of encapsulating peritoneal sclerosis. This in addition to technique failure can result in morbidity (bowel obstruction, malnutrition) as well as mortality [3]. Understanding the unique risk factors for peritonitis in children and the challenges associated with the management is necessary to take adequate steps for the prevention of peritonitis.

In this chapter, we review the challenges with peritonitis in children on chronic PD.

14.2 Difficult-to-Treat Peritonitis

14.2.1 Relapsing Peritonitis

The ISPD guidelines define two or more episodes of peritonitis as recurrent, relapsing or repeat depending on the timing and the organism causing peritonitis [4]. The definitions are stated in Table 14.1. Peritonitis that occurs within 4 weeks of completion of therapy for peritonitis with the same organism of a culture-negative peritonitis is defined as relapsing peritonitis. Recurrent peritonitis is defined as peritonitis that occurs within 4 weeks of completion of therapy for a prior episode of peritonitis but with a different organism. Repeat peritonitis occurs beyond 4 weeks of completion of therapy. If peritonitis is caused by the same organism, it is called repeat peritonitis; if it is by a different organism, it is defined as re-infection.

Relapsing peritonitis can be difficult to treat and may result in catheter removal and reduced function of the peritoneal membrane [5, 6]. Relapsing peritonitis has been documented in 5–20% of peritonitis in data from adults and children [7, 8].

Data from the International paediatric peritoneal dialysis network (IPPN) showed in comparison to other studies, the incidence of recurrent peritonitis was higher with peritonitis secondary to *S. aureus* and Gram-negative organisms. Culture-negative peritonitis relapsing peritonitis had a poor response to therapy. Younger age, single cuff catheter and chronic systemic antibiotic prophylaxis were significant risk factors. Relapsing peritonitis was associated with a higher risk of ultrafiltration failure, full functional recovery and technique failure [9].

Table 14.1 Definitions for peritonitis beyond the first episode

Duration since completion of treatment for first episode	Same organism	Different organism
<4 weeks	Relapse	Recurrent
>4 weeks	Repeat	Re-infection

Treatment—Relapsing peritonitis is associated with a high risk of membrane damage and technique failure. Hence early intervention is crucial. Antibiotic therapy based on the previous culture sensitivity may be initiated till the culture reports are available. If methicillin-resistant *S. aureus* is suspected, vancomycin should be given in addition to Gram-negative coverage. The guidelines recommend antibiotic therapy for 3 weeks in the case of relapsing peritonitis. The cure rate following antibiotic therapy for relapsing peritonitis has been found to be around 75% in both adult and paediatric studies [10].

There is some data from adult studies to show the benefits of intraluminal urokinase instillation on early resolution and prevention of relapse. However, in the absence of data from paediatric studies, instillation of a thrombolytic agent is not routinely recommended in children [10]. Data from the IPPN [9] as well as from adult and paediatric patients from the ANZDATA registry [11] show that relapsing peritonitis in comparison to sporadic peritonitis have a higher rate of technique failure and change of dialysis modality.

Catheter removal is indicated as soon as the infection is controlled in case of relapsing peritonitis associated with exit site or tunnel infection or second relapse. Simultaneous re-insertion of a new catheter is recommended to obviate the need for temporary hemodialysis.

14.2.2 Fungal Peritonitis

Fungal peritonitis is a rare but serious complication in children on peritoneal dialysis. The incidence of fungal peritonitis ranges from 2 to 10% in the paediatric PD population. Fungal peritonitis is associated with a higher risk of membrane and technique failure as well as mortality. The initial data on fungal peritonitis in children was reported from the NAPRTCS database in the early 1990s. However, during this period of time, the definitions of peritonitis were not established by the ISPD guidelines. Also, a majority of children during that time had a single cuff catheter and were on continuous ambulatory peritoneal dialysis [12].

More recently, retrospective multi-centre data from the Netherlands showed that the prevalence of fungal peritonitis was 2.9%. *Candida* was the most common organism isolated. Higher bacterial peritonitis rate, peritonitis with Gram-negative organisms and recent use of antibiotics were all risk factors for fungal peritonitis [13].

A study comparing the worldwide variation in peritonitis found that the overall incidence of fungal peritonitis was around 3% and was comparable between different regions [14].

A study from Iran found that relapsing peritonitis and administration of antibiotics in the last 1 month before the episode of fungal peritonitis were important risk factors. Fungal peritonitis was associated with catheter malfunction and was also associated with an increased like of mortality [15].

A large retrospective cohort from China showed that *Candida parapsilosis* was the most common organism. All patients with fungal peritonitis were switched to haemodialysis and did not return to PD. In the multivariate analysis, they found that lower serum albumin was a risk factor for fungal peritonitis [16].

In contrast, a larger cohort of children from the SCOPE collaborative showed that the prevalence of fungal peritonitis was about 8%; with fungal peritonitis being the first episode of peritonitis in about half of the cohort. Only 17% of children had previous bacterial peritonitis in the preceding 1 month. Children <2 years of age had a higher risk for fungal peritonitis when compared to older children. When compared to other causes of peritonitis, fungal peritonitis was associated with a longer duration of hospitalisation, increased rate of catheter removal and higher risk of technique failure [17].

14.2.3 Culture Negative Peritonitis

The ISPD guidelines [4] recommend that the culture-negative peritonitis rates should ideally be <15%. A failure to achieve the recommended rate should prompt a review of the protocols for sample collection and processing.

The analysis of data from the IPPN looking at the worldwide variation in peritonitis showed that the overall incidence of culture-negative peritonitis was 29% [7]. Other studies have reported rates varying from 11 to 67% [18].

The SCOPE collaborative studied culture-negative peritonitis rates across various centres. The ISPD guidelines for centrifugation of the effluent before inoculation was not followed in more than 50% of centres. The culture media used, use of BACTEC and PCR techniques were varied. In contrast to adult data which showed that larger centres with a higher number of peritoneal dialysis catheters had a lower culture-negative rate, the incidence of culture-negative peritonitis was not affected by the size of the centre for paediatric dialysis. Though centres that had patients performing their own dialysis without an adult caregiver had a higher rate of culture-negative peritonitis than those with an adult caregiver, the median age at first peritonitis was not significantly different. Samples obtained after a shorter dwell had a lower white cell count and a higher rate of negative culture. The protocols for sample collection and processing did not have a significant impact on the rate of culture-negative peritonitis rate. The outcome was culture-negative peritonitis was good probably due to prompt initiation of suitable antibiotics. The favourable outcome also implies that culture-negative peritonitis is unlikely to be due to non-infectious causes or atypical organisms as is often reported in the adult population. To increase the rate of detecting organisms, the SCOPE collaborative used the PD fluid culture bundle [18].

The outcomes of peritonitis in children from the IPPN registry showed that culture-negative peritonitis had a favourable rate of recovery, technique failure and relapse rate when compared to culture-positive peritonitis [19].

14.3 PD Catheter and Peritonitis

14.3.1 Catheter Leak

Catheter leaks are a common non-infectious complication of peritoneal dialysis that can lead to peritonitis. Figure 14.1 demonstrates the leak of dialysate fluid from the pericatheter site in a child with nephrotic syndrome. The leak may be to the exterior or into the subcutaneous plane. Rarely, the leaks may cause hydrothorax or genital edema. Early break-in, large dwell volume, use of single cuff catheters predisposes to catheter leaks. Leaks may be managed conservatively with peritoneal rest, switch to haemodialysis if necessary and use of lower dwell volumes. Fibrin glue has been tried with success in some cases [20].

14.3.2 Cuff Extrusion

There is limited literature on the prevalence and risk factors for cuff extrusion in children as well as adults with chronic PD. Figure 14.2 demonstrates cuff extrusion in an infant with severe malnutrition. It is a well-known risk factor for peritonitis and exit site infection and should be looked for in every child with peritonitis. A case series of recurrent exit site infections due to *S. aureus* associated with cuff extrusion has been reported. Cuff shaving reduced the risk of exit site infections.

The proposed risk factors for cuff extrusion are inappropriate placement of the external cuff in the skin rather than in the fat plane or a reduced fat plane as seen in neonates/young infants, malnourished children and abdominal wall abnormalities like Prune belly syndrome. It may also occur with an exit site infection.

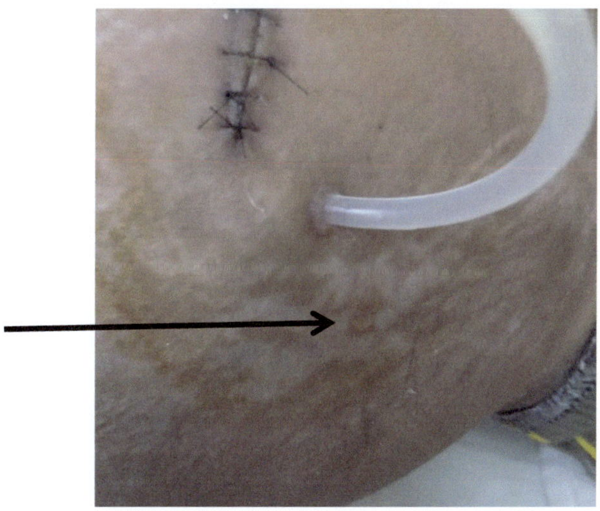

Fig. 14.1 Leak from the pericatheter site in a child with nephrotic syndrome and severe ascites and abdominal wall edema

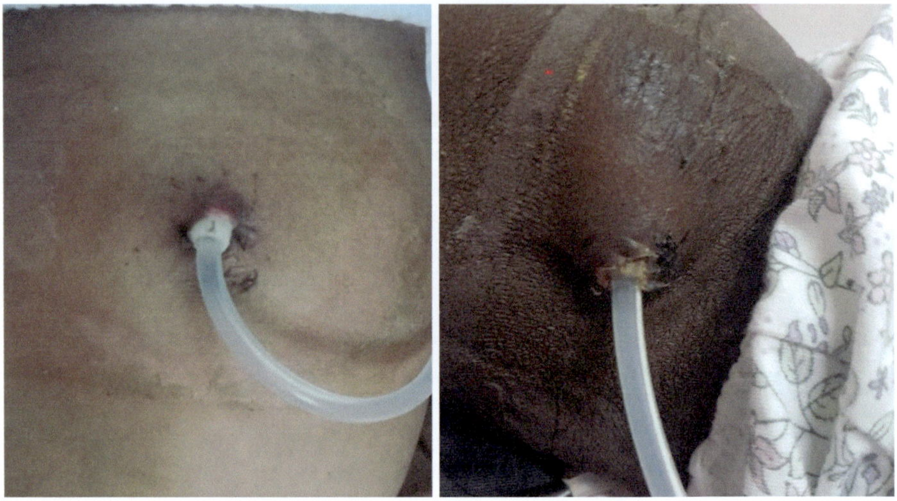

Fig. 14.2 Cuff extrusion in infants with kidney failure and severe malnutrition

Shaving of the superficial cuff can be done in cases with cuff extrusion. If symptoms persist, catheter replacement is recommended [20].

14.3.3 Hole in the Catheter

Breach in the peritoneal dialysis catheter, as well as catheter handling, is a major risk factor for peritonitis. The hole in the catheter with leak of dialysate is shown in Fig. 14.3. Accidental touch contamination is known to predispose to peritonitis and the ISPD guidelines [4] recommend a change of the transfer set and prophylactic antibiotics along with close observation for the occurrence of peritonitis. A hole in the catheter through an uncommon complication has been associated with peritonitis. When looking for plausible causes of peritonitis in children on chronic dialysis, data from the IPPN registry showed that touch contamination was reported as a cause in 12% and a hole in the catheter was reported in 2% of children with a known risk factor for peritonitis [19].

Catheter breakage may occur due to a faulty adapter, due to the natural wear and tear process, following prolonged use of catheter repeated contact with chemicals like disinfectants, mupirocin etc., use of sharp objects like scissors during dressing or sharp clamps. A study in a paediatric cohort showed that the rate of transfer set holes was higher than accidental exposures/touch contamination. There was a trend of higher WBC count with the holes in the catheter. All children with holes or accidental exposure receive prophylactic antibiotics and the rate of peritonitis was low [21].

In case of a distal hole, the catheter may be cut proximally. If the hole is close to the exit site, it requires replacement of the catheter.

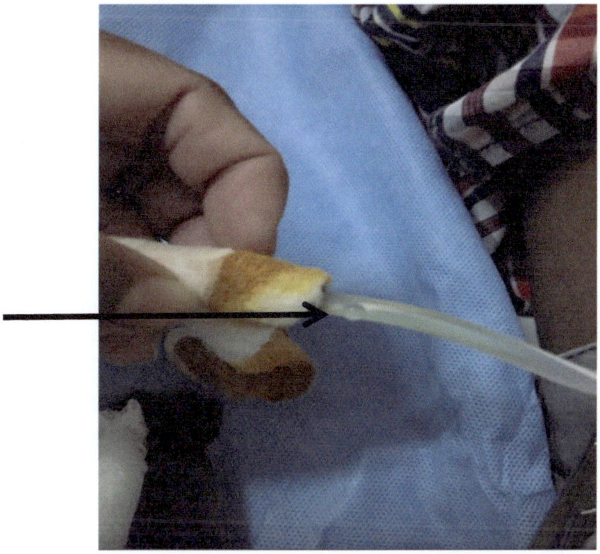

Fig. 14.3 Hole in the peritoneal dialysis catheter with leak of dialysate

14.4 Other Unique Risk Factors for Peritonitis in Children

14.4.1 Stomas and Peritonitis

Gastrostomy is an important modality to administer nutritional supplementation to infants and young children on dialysis. A relationship between percutaneous gastrostomy and fungal peritonitis has been reported in some studies. Data from the IPPN registry showed an association of Gram-negative peritonitis with gastrostomy [19].

However, more recent studies have failed to demonstrate an increased risk of peritonitis with gastrostomy. A laparoscopic or open gastrostomy may be recommended for children already on PD or initiating PD in the near future.

In contrast, data from the IPPN registry showed that in children with a colostomy, though chronic PD is a feasible option, it is associated with a higher risk of peritonitis and exit site infections when compared to the control group. There was also a higher incidence of mortality [22].

14.4.2 Ventriculo-Peritoneal (VP) Shunts and Peritonitis

In a case series reported from the IPPN database, peritoneal dialysis was feasible and safe in children with VP shunts with no increased risk of ascending or descending infections [23].

14.4.3 PD in Infants

Though PD is the preferred and, in some settings the only modality for renal replacement therapy in infants with kidney failure, the challenges of PD in this cohort are many. The clinical practice guidelines for the management of infants with kidney failure emphasise on the high risk of infections, the risk factors and outcomes [24].

Young age is an important risk factor for peritonitis. The NAPRTCS data showed that the annualised rate of peritonitis was much higher in infants when compared to older children [25].

More recent data from the SCOPE collaborative also suggests a high annualised rate of peritonitis in infants, with especially higher rates in the initial period after catheter placement [26].

The common risk factors associated with peritonitis like cuff extrusion, catheter leakage due to weak abdominal wall or malnutrition, exit site tunnel infection and presence of a stoma/gastrostomy are likely to be more common in infants than in older children. The SCOPE collaborative also found that the need for nephrectomy and placement of a gastrostomy were associated with an increased risk of peritonitis.

The NAPRTCS data also showed that the rate of hospitalisations was higher in infants on PD when compared to older children. Similarly, the SCOPE collaborative also showed that infants of PD with peritonitis had higher morbidity and longer duration of hospitalisation [27].

14.4.4 Challenges with PD in Low-Resource Countries

The challenges of performing peritoneal dialysis in low-resource settings are several. The low educational level of caregivers, poor housing conditions and lack of clean water supply are some of the problems that may hinder optimal dialysis training and performance. In addition, lack of financial support, high out-of-pocket expenses and large distance from health care centre are impediments to regular follow-up and monitoring. In a study from our centre on PD in low body weight children, we emphasised the challenges in providing optimal care for children on PD. [28]

14.4.5 Encapsulating Peritoneal Sclerosis (EPS)

EPS is a rare but serious complication of chronic peritoneal dialysis. Though rarely reported in children, it can be a significant cause of morbidity and mortality. The time on peritoneal dialysis, use of conventional non-biocompatible dialysate and multiple episodes of peritonitis are proposed risk factors for EPS in children [29].

14.4.6 Caregiver Burden

Caregiver burden is an important aspect to be considered in the care of children on chronic peritoneal dialysis. Studies have shown that managing a child on chronic peritoneal dialysis and its complications like peritonitis can impose physical, psychological, social and financial burdens on the caregivers as well as other members of the family [30]. These aspects must be addressed to ensure holistic care for a child on chronic dialysis.

Important Points

- Difficult-to-treat peritonitis as seen in relapsing, recurrent or fungal peritonitis are an important cause of morbidity and technique failure.
- PD access itself can be an important cause of peritonitis and protocols for insertion and management of PD access issues are important to prevent peritonitis.
- Unique situations needing individualised management are infant dialysis, presence of stomas/shunts and caregiver burden, especially where automated PD is not feasible.
- Peritonitis can have devastating consequences resulting in membrane failure and care must be taken to prevent peritonitis in all children on peritoneal dialysis.

References

1. North American Pediatric Renal Trials and Collaborative Studies (NAPRTCS) 2011 annual dialysis report. Available at: https://web.emmes.com/study/ped/annlrept/annualrept2011.pdf
2. United States Renal Data System (USRDS) 2013 report. Available at: http://www.usrds.org/2013/pdf/v2_ch8_13.pdf
3. Shroff R, Stefanidis CJ, Askiti V, Edefonti A, Testa S, Ekim M, et al. Encapsulating peritoneal sclerosis in children on chronic PD: a survey from the European paediatric dialysis working group. Nephrol Dial Transplant. 2013;28:1908–14.
4. Li PK, Chow KM, Cho Y, Fan S, Figueiredo AE, Harris T, et al. ISPD peritonitis guideline recommendations: 2022 update on prevention and treatment. Perit Dial Int. 2022;42:110–53.
5. Klaus G, Schaefer F, Querfeld U, Soergel M, Wolf S, Mehls A. Treatment of relapsing peritonitis in pediatric patients on peritoneal dialysis. Adv Perit Dial. 1992;8:302–5.
6. Andreoli SP, Leiser J, Warady BA, Schlichting L, Brewer ED. Adverse effect of peritonitis on peritoneal membrane function in children on dialysis. Pediatr Nephrol. 1999;13:1–6.
7. Schaefer F, Feneberg R, Aksu N, Donmez O, Sadikoglu B, Alexander SR, et al. Worldwide variation of dialysisassociated peritonitis in children. Kidney Int. 2007;72:1374–9.
8. Burke M, Hawley CM, Badve SV, McDonald SP, Brown FG, Boudville N, et al. Relapsing and recurrent peritoneal dialysis-associated peritonitis: a multicenter registry study. Am J Kidney Dis. 2011;58:429–36.
9. Lane JC, Warady BA, Feneberg R, Majkowski NL, Watson AR, Fischbach M, et al. International pediatric peritonitis Registry. Relapsing peritonitis in children who undergo chronic peritoneal dialysis: a prospective study of the international pediatric peritonitis registry. Clin J Am Soc Nephrol. 2010;5:1041–6.

10. Bakkaloglu SA, Warady BA. Difficult peritonitis cases in children undergoing chronic peritoneal dialysis: relapsing, repeat, recurrent and zoonotic episodes. Pediatr Nephrol. 2015;30:1397–406.
11. Bordador EB, Johnson DW, Henning P, Kennedy SE, McDonald SP, Burke JR, et al. Australian and New Zealand Dialysis andTransplant Registry. Epidemiology and outcomes of peritonitis in children on peritoneal dialysis in Australasia. Pediatr Nephrol. 2010;25:1739–45.
12. Warady BA, Bashir M, Donaldson LA. Fungal peritonitis in children receiving peritoneal dialysis: a report of the NAPRTCS. Kidney Int. 2000;58:384–9.
13. Raaijmakers R, Schröder C, Monnens L, Cornelissen E, Warris A. Fungal peritonitis in children on peritoneal dialysis. Pediatr Nephrol. 2007;22:288–93.
14. Schaefer F, Feneberg R, Aksu N, Donmez O, Sadikoglu B, Alexander SR, et al. Worldwide variation of dialysis-associated peritonitis in children. Kidney Int. 2007;72:1374–9.
15. Hooman N, Madani A, Sharifian Dorcheh M, Mahdavi A, Derakhshan A, Gheissari A, et al. Fungal peritonitis in Iranian children on continuous ambulatory peritoneal dialysis: a national experience. Iran J Kidney Dis. 2007;1:29–33.
16. Fang X, Cui J, Zhai Y, Liu J, Rao J, Zhang Z, et al. Clinical features and risk factors of fungal peritonitis in children on peritoneal dialysis. Front Pediatr. 2021;30(9):683992.
17. Munshi R, Sethna CB, Richardson T, Rodean J, Al-Akash S, Gupta S, et al. Fungal peritonitis in the standardizing care to improve outcomes in pediatric end stage renal disease (SCOPE) collaborative. Pediatr Nephrol. 2018;33:873–80.
18. Davis TK, Bryant KA, Rodean J, Richardson T, Selvarangan R, Qin X, et al. Variability in culture-negative peritonitis rates in pediatric peritoneal Dialysis programs in the United States. Clin J Am Soc Nephrol. 2021;16:233–40.
19. Warady BA, Feneberg R, Verrina E, Flynn JT, Müller-Wiefel DE, Besbas N, et al. IPPR. Peritonitis in children who receive long-term peritoneal dialysis: a prospective evaluation of therapeutic guidelines. J Am Soc Nephrol. 2007;18:2172–9.
20. Fraser N, Hussain FK, Connell R, Shenoy MU. Chronic peritoneal dialysis in children. Int J Nephrol Renovasc Dis. 2015;8:125–37.
21. Silverstein DM, Wilcox JE. Outcome of accidental peritoneal dialysis catheter holes or tip exposure. Pediatr Nephrol. 2010;25:1147–51.
22. Chan EYH, Borzych-Duzalka D, Alparslan C, Harvey E, Munarriz RL, Runowski D, et al. International pediatric peritoneal Dialysis network Colostomy in children on chronic peritoneal dialysis. Pediatr Nephrol. 2020;35:119–26.
23. Dolan NM, Borzych-Duzalka D, Suarez A, Principi I, Hernandez O, Al-Akash S, et al. Ventriculoperitoneal shunts in children on peritoneal dialysis: a survey of the international pediatric peritoneal Dialysis network. Pediatr Nephrol. 2013;28:315–9.
24. Zurowska AM, Fischbach M, Watson AR, Edefonti A, Stefanidis CJ. European Paediatric Dialysis working group. Clinical practice recommendations for the care of infants with stage 5 chronic kidney disease (CKD5). Pediatr Nephrol. 2013;28:1739–48.
25. North American Pediatric Renal Trials and Collaborative Studies (NAPRTCS). 2014 Annual Dialysis Report. Available at: https://web.emmes.com/study/ped/annlrept/annualrept2014.pdf
26. Zaritsky JJ, Hanevold C, Quigley R, Richardson T, Wong C, Ehrlich J, et al. Epidemiology of peritonitis following maintenance peritoneal dialysis catheter placement during infancy: a report of the SCOPE collaborative. Pediatr Nephrol. 2018;33:713–22.
27. Niang A, Iyengar A, Luyckx VA. Hemodialysis versus peritoneal dialysis in resource-limited settings. Curr Opin Nephrol Hypertens. 2018;27:463–71.
28. Kamath N, Reddy HV, Iyengar A. Clinical and dialysis outcomes of manual chronic peritoneal dialysis in low-body-weight children from a low-to-middle-income country. Perit Dial Int. 2020;40:6–11.
29. Stefanidis CJ, Shroff R. Encapsulating peritoneal sclerosis in children. Pediatr Nephrol. 2014;29:2093–103.
30. Wightman A. Caregiver burden in pediatric dialysis. Pediatr Nephrol. 2020;35:1575–83.

MIX
Papier aus verantwortungsvollen Quellen
Paper from responsible sources
FSC® C105338

If you have any concerns about our products,
you can contact us on
ProductSafety@springernature.com

In case Publisher is established outside the EU,
the EU authorized representative is:
Springer Nature Customer Service Center GmbH
Europaplatz 3, 69115 Heidelberg, Germany

Printed by Libri Plureos GmbH
in Hamburg, Germany